U0325211

ABC of
Quality Improvement
in Healthcare

ABC 医疗质量改进

著 者 [英] 蒂姆·斯旺威克 (Tim Swanwick)

[英] 艾玛·沃克斯 (Emma Vaux)

主 译 唐惠君 孙 杰 刘西纺

WILEY

 湖南科学技术出版社

·长沙·

图书在版编目（ＣＩＰ）数据

ABC医疗质量改进 / (英) 蒂姆·斯旺威克, (英) 艾玛·沃克斯著; 唐惠君, 孙杰, 刘西纺主译. —长沙: 湖南科学技术出版社, 2023.3
（全科医学系列丛书）
ISBN 978-7-5710-1868-9

Ⅰ. ①A… Ⅱ. ①蒂… ②艾… ③唐… ④孙… ⑤刘… Ⅲ. ①医疗质量管理 Ⅳ. ①R197.323.4

中国版本图书馆 CIP 数据核字 (2022) 第 210270 号

ABC YILIAO ZHILIANG GAIJIN
ABC 医疗质量改进

著　　者：[英] 蒂姆·斯旺威克　[英] 艾玛·沃克斯
主　　译：唐惠君　孙　杰　刘西纺
出 版 人：潘晓山
出版统筹：张忠丽
责任编辑：李　忠
文字编辑：白汀竹
特约编辑：王超萍
出版发行：湖南科学技术出版社
社　　址：长沙市芙蓉中路一段 416 号泊富国际金融中心
网　　址：http://www.hnstp.com
湖南科学技术出版社天猫旗舰店网址：
　　　　　http://hnkjcbs.tmall.com
邮购联系：0731-84375808
印　　刷：湖南凌宇纸品有限公司
　　　　　（印装质量问题请直接与本厂联系）
厂　　址：长沙县黄花镇黄垅新村工业园财富大道16号
邮　　编：410137
版　　次：2023 年 3 月第 1 版
印　　次：2023 年 3 月第 1 次印刷
开　　本：787mm×1092mm　1/16
印　　张：9.25
字　　数：219 千字
书　　号：ISBN 978-7-5710-1868-9
定　　价：99.00 元
（版权所有·翻印必究）

List of Translators

译者委员会

主　译　唐惠君　惠州卫生职业技术学院附属医院

　　　　　孙　杰　宁波市第一医院

　　　　　刘西纺　西安交通大学附属红会医院

副主译　杨荣华　广州市第一人民医院

　　　　　金　静　四川省人民医院

　　　　　田　竞　中国人民解放军北部战区总医院

　　　　　林锦波　香港中文大学（深圳）附属第二医院 /
　　　　　　　　　深圳市龙岗区人民医院

译　者　张　霆　上海中医药大学附属龙华医院

　　　　　曾昭宇　成都市第三人民医院

　　　　　田　竞　中国人民解放军北部战区总医院

　　　　　姚　蕾　武汉科技大学附属老年病医院

　　　　　郝又国　同济大学附属普陀人民医院

　　　　　苏跃康　个旧市人民医院

　　　　　郝书理　香港中文大学（深圳）附属第二医院 /
　　　　　　　　　深圳市龙岗区人民医院

　　　　　张晓燕　香港中文大学（深圳）附属第二医院 /
　　　　　　　　　深圳市龙岗区人民医院

Preface

前　言

Written and edited by some of the leading practitioners in the field, the ABC of Quality Improvement in Healthcare attempts to demystify quality improvement, providing comprehensive coverage and clear and succinct descriptions of the major tools, techniques and approaches used in this emerging discipline.

The ABC of Quality Improvement in Healthcare is designed for clinicians new to the field as well as for experienced leaders of change and improvement. It will be relevant to doctors, dentists, nurses and other healthcare professionals at various levels, as well as to health service managers and support staff. The book is particularly appropriate for guiding medical students and doctors in training and their tutors and trainers.

After reading the ABC of Quality Improvement in Healthcare readers will not only have a broad understanding of what constitutes quality in healthcare but also how to measure it, design improvement interventions that really make a difference and manage change projects within their own organisations. Practical examples will be provided along the way and readers signposted to a host of useful resources. Tips for successful projects will be highlighted alongside some of the common pitfalls. Above anything, the ABC of Quality Improvement in Healthcare will give readers the confidence to embark on their own improvement projects, whoever and wherever they may be. We hope you will find it useful.

Tim Swanwick
Emma Vaux

《ABC 医疗质量改进》由该领域的一些专家编写，全面、清晰、简洁地描述了这一新兴学科中使用的主要工具、技术和方法，试图揭开质量改进的神秘面纱。

本书为初次接触该领域的临床医生以及有经验的变革和改进领导者编写，医生、牙医、护士和其他各级医疗专业人员以及医疗服务管理和支持人员均可使用。本书极其适合做培训教材，不仅可以用于医学生和医生的培训，也可供指导教师和培训师参考。

阅读本书后，读者不仅会对医疗保健质量的构成有全面的了解，而且还将掌握评价体系，施行有益的改进措施，并在自己的领域内管理改进项目。我们将在此过程中提供一些实用的案例，并为读者提供许多为之受益的资源。项目成功的要点与一些常见的陷阱并列突出显示。最重要的是，《ABC 医疗质量改进》会让读者拥有信心，让他们无论身在何处，都能开始自己的改进项目。我们希望你能从本书中获得助益。

蒂姆·斯旺威克
艾玛·沃克斯

Contents

目　录

Tim Swanwick[1] *and Emma Vaux*[2]

[1] Director, Clinical Leadership Development, NHS Leadership Academy, NHS England and NHS Improvement, Leeds, UK
[2] Consultant nephrologist and general physician, Royal Berkshire NHS Foundation Trust; Vice President for Education and Training, Royal College of Physicians (RCP), London, UK

OVERVIEW
概述

- Quality is the degree of excellence of something; how good or bad it is.
  质量用于描述事物的卓越程度，多好或多差。
- Quality in healthcare describes the degree to which care is safe, effective and provides a good patient experience.
  医疗质量描述了医疗安全、有效和提供良好患者体验的程度。
- Quality can be measured in terms of structures, processes and outcomes.
  质量可以根据结构、过程和结果来衡量。
- Value-based approaches go beyond quality to consider population health outcomes and what really matters to patients.
  比质量更重要的是价值，即需要考虑人口的健康以及患者真正重要的事情。

What is quality?

Quality is an elusive concept, not helped by the way we commonly use the word in the English language. Quality can mean the extent to which something meets a standard or set of standards. So, healthcare may be of high or low *quality*. But it can also refer to a distinguishing characteristic or property possessed by something – among the qualities of this book for instance, is that it is brief and to the point – or even as a synonym for excellence; it is, of course, a *quality* publication. For the remainder of the book we will adopt the first of these as our general definition, that is quality as the degree of excellence of something; how good or bad it is.

什么是质量

"质量"是一个难以捉摸的概念，在英语中这个词通常无助于理解。质量可以是指某物达到一个标准或一组标准的程度。因此，医疗可能是高质量的，也可能是低质量的。但它也可以指某事物所具有的显著特征或属性——例如，在本书中所言的质量，它是简明扼要的，甚至是卓越的同义词；当然，这是一本高质量的出版物。在本书的其余部分，将采用上述第一个作为一般定义，即质量用于描述某事物的卓越程度，即有多好或有多不好。

This then, immediately raises a question about the dimensions of 'excellence' that we are interested in. What specifically in healthcare is important to us, that we would wish to set standards, measure and seek to improve?

Quality in healthcare

In 1999, the US Institute of Medicine published the first of a series of outputs from its project The Quality of Health Care in America. *To Err is Human* (Kohn et al., 2000) was a wake-up call, full of shocking statistics about medical error and the disparity between the incidence of such errors and public perception of the infallibility of the healthcare professions. The follow-up publication, *Crossing the Quality Chasm* (Committee on Quality of Health Care in America, Institute of Medicine, 2001), was more forward looking and proposed a strategic framework for quality improvement in healthcare. Contained within the report is a statement of purpose for those who seek to improve healthcare quality: to bring about 'improved health, greater longevity, less pain and suffering, and increased personal productivity to those who receive their care'.

The Institute of Medicine went on to describe six 'aims', effectively domains that describe the areas to which we need to attend when considering the quality of healthcare (Figure 1.1). These are the extent to which healthcare is:

然后，这立即提出一个问题，即卓越的维度。在医疗领域，对我们来说什么是重要的，以至于我们希望制定标准、措施并寻求改进。

医疗质量

1999 年，美国医学研究所发表了《错误在人》（Kohn 等，2000 年），这篇文章是其项目 "美国医疗质量" 系列成果的第一篇。它敲响了警钟，里面展示了骇人的医疗事故统计数据，并且公众对医疗行业越信任，此类事故的发生率就越高。后续出版的《跨越质量鸿沟》（美国医疗质量委员会、医学研究所，2001 年）更具前瞻性，提出了医疗质量改进的战略框架。报告中包含了一份旨在改进医疗质量的声明：为那些接受护理的人 "改善健康、延长寿命、减少疼痛和痛苦并提高个人生产力"。

医学研究所接着描述了 6 个目标，有效地描述了在考虑医疗质量时需要关注的领域（图 1.1）。这些是医疗质量的范围：

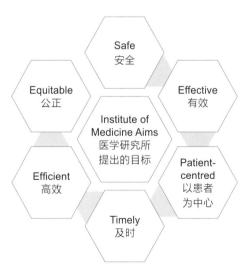

Figure 1.1 Six domains of healthcare quality. Source: Institute of Medicine.

图 1.1 医疗质量的 6 个领域。资料来源：医学研究所

Safe: avoiding injuries to patients from the care that is intended to help them.

Effective: providing services based on scientific knowledge to all who could benefit, and refraining from providing services to those not likely to benefit.

Patient-centred: providing care that is respectful of and responsive to individual patient preferences, needs and values, and ensuring that patient values guide all clinical decisions.

Timely: reducing waits and sometimes harmful delays for both those who receive and those who give care.

Efficient: avoiding waste, including waste of equipment, supplies, ideas and energy.

Equitable: providing care that does not vary in quality because of personal characteristics such as gender, ethnicity, geographic location and socioeconomic status.

Similar lists can be found throughout the world; indeed, the World Health Organisation adopts an almost identical definition of the quality of care: 'the extent to which health care services provided to individuals and patient populations improve desired health outcomes. In order to achieve this, health care must be safe, effective, timely, efficient, equitable and people-centred' (WHO, 2016). And the NHS in England has a similar outlook on quality, namely that it should be safe, 'effective and provide a positive patient experience' (NHS, 2016).

Measuring quality

When it comes to assessing quality within the above domains, we have a number of options about what we choose to measure. Donabedian provides a useful conceptual model for examining services and evaluating quality of healthcare. According to Donabedian (1966), information about quality of care can be drawn from three categories: 'structure', 'process' and 'outcomes'.

Structure describes the context in which care is delivered. This might include the equipment used, the staff available and the buildings in which care takes place. Staffing ratios on wards are a structural measure of quality.

Process refers to the interactions between patients and staff, and between staff themselves, during the delivery of an intervention or

安全：避免患者受到护理活动的伤害，尽管这些护理措施的出发点是好的。

有效：向所有可能受益的人提供科学服务，避免向不太可能受益的人提供服务。

以患者为中心：提供尊重和契合患者个人偏好、需求和价值观的护理，并确保患者价值观指导所有临床决策。

及时：减少患者和照顾者的等待时间或延误。

高效：避免浪费，包括浪费设备、用品、决策和能源。

公平：无论患者的性别、民族、所在地理位置和社会经济地位等如何，均提供质量不变的护理。

世界各地都可以找到类似的清单。事实上，世界卫生组织对护理质量采取了几乎与本书相同的定义："向世人提供能达到其预期治疗效果的医疗服务水平。为了实现这一目标，医疗保健活动必须安全、有效、及时、高效、公平和以人为本"（WHO，2016 年）。英国国家医疗服务体系（NHS）对质量也有类似的看法，即应该安全，"有效并提供良好的患者体验"（NHS，2016）。

质量的测量

在评估上述领域内的质量时，有很多可供评估的内容。多纳贝迪安为检查服务水平和评估医疗质量提供了有用的概念模式。根据多纳贝迪安的说法（1966 年），护理质量可从"结构""流程"和"结果"3 个类别进行评估。

"结构"用于描述护理环境。这包括所使用的设备、可用的工作人员以及护理病房状况。病房的人员配置比率是测量质量的结构性指标。

"流程"是指在实施干预措施或护理时，患者与员工之间以及员工之间的互动过程。

an episode of care. An example might be the frequency that a deteriorating patient is reviewed.

Finally, *outcomes* are the manifestations of the effects of healthcare interventions on the health and well-being of patients and populations. This could include anything from institutional mortality rates to population-based measures of well-being.

Quality control, assurance and improvement

We have three further definitions to explore before proceeding: quality control, quality assurance and (the subject of this book) quality improvement.

Quality control is an internal process designed to compare the level of performance of a system against adopted standards or benchmarks. It should be continual, responsive and used by people closest to, and responsible for, the work. An example might be the repeated checking of results in the biomedical laboratory where statistical processes are used to monitor the reliability of machines and processes that produce patient blood results.

Quality assurance also evaluates performance; it is the planned and systematic process of gathering evidence to provide confidence that a system is meeting internal or external standards. Assurance is measured after the event. As an example of quality assurance in relation to the example given above, laboratory staff would periodically perform audits to check the number of errors occurring. This provides information on whether an acceptable level of safety is being achieved.

Quality assurance is an essential part of good governance, where boards or governing bodies will seek evidence-based 'assurance', rather than reassurance. Evidence commonly used by hospital boards as part of quality assurance processes includes achievement of nationally approved standards and targets, clinical incident reporting, patient surveys and number of complaints, staff surveys and mortality rate. This is often combined with the process of identifying good practice, as well as that which falls below standard, and the publication or dissemination of results. Similar information on care quality is also sought by commissioners and regulators

一个可能发生的例子是，复查频繁致患者病情恶化。

最后，"结果"是医疗干预对患者和大众健康和福祉的影响。这包括住院死亡率、某地区人口的幸福指数等。

质量控制、保证和改进

在继续论述之前，我们还有 3 个定义要探讨：质量控制、质量保证和质量改进（本书的主题）。

质量控制是一个内部过程，旨在将系统的性能水平与采用的标准或基准进行比较。它应该不断持续并对问题及时响应，并由专人负责这项工作。以生物医学实验室对化验结果的重复检查为例，其中的统计过程用于监控得出患者血液化验结果的机器及其检测过程是否可靠。

质量保证也评估效果，这是有计划和系统地收集证据的过程，目的是确保系统满足内部或外部标准，而且需要事后测量。举个与上个例子相关的例子，实验室工作人员将定期按表格进行审查，通过核实错误数量来判断是否达到安全级别。

质量保证是良好治理的重要组成部分，董事会或管理机构将以证据为基础，而不是想象。在这个过程中，医院董事会通常认可的证据包括国家批准的标准和目标、临床事件报告、患者调查和投诉数量、员工调查和死亡率。这通常需要制定实践标准以及及时公布调查结果。监管机构也在寻求类似的护理质量信息，从而导致了"担保"行业的蓬勃发展。

resulting, in many instances, in a burgeoning assurance 'industry'.

Quality improvement describes a systematic process to improve quality; areas are identified for improvement, the problem understood, solutions tested and the impact of any change evaluated and measured. An example might be improving waiting times to access a mental health service, reducing the length of stay and bed occupancy or reducingmedication error in the emergency department. There is no single definition of quality improvement, and no one approach appears to be more successful than another. Quality improvement, or QI for short, is explored in detail in the chapters that follow.

Theories of quality

For those wishing to explore the theories that surround the concept of 'quality' and its management we have provided signposts to some further reading. But before moving on it is worth pausing briefly to reflect on the work of a handful of significant and influential 'quality' thinkers:

Joseph Juran (1904–2008) was a passionate advocate for quality management both in the US and Japan. He is best known for his 'quality trilogy' distinguishing between quality planning, control and improvement, and his adoption and promulgation of the Pareto principle; that 80% of the problems are produced by 20% of the causes (see Chapter 8). Juran identified 10 steps to quality improvement and emphasised that if a quality improvement project is to be successful, then all quality improvement actions must be carefully planned out and controlled.

W. Edwards Deming (1900–1993) also made a significant contribution to the quality practices of the post-war Japanese and US manufacturing industries. Alongside Phillip Crosby (1926–2001) he is credited with being the father of Total Quality Management (TQM) and developed his own 14 principles of improvement. The culmination of his work was though his System of Profound Knowledge, which serves to highlight that if we really want to make improvement progress in the messiness of real world we need to consider four broad domains:

- appreciation of a system
- knowledge of variation

质量改进描述了提高质量的系统过程，包括确定改进领域、理解问题、测试解决方案以及评估和考查变革带来的影响。例如，缩短心理健康服务的等待时间、减少住院时间和床位占用或减少急诊室的用药失误。质量改进没有唯一的定义，也没有哪种方法最好。随后的章节将详细探讨质量改进（QI）。

质量理论

对于那些希望探索质量的概念及其管理理论的人，我们提供了进一步阅读的清单。但在继续讨论之前，有必要暂停一会儿，回顾一下少数有影响力的质量研究者的工作：

约瑟夫·朱兰（1904—2008 年）曾是美国和日本质量管理体系的积极倡导者。其最著名的是"质量三部曲"——区分了质量计划、控制和改进。他采纳并应用了帕累托原则，即 80% 的问题是由 20% 的原因造成的（见第 8 章）。朱兰确定了质量改进的 10 个步骤，并强调质量改进项目要成功，那么所有的质量改进步骤都必须仔细规划和控制。

爱德华兹·戴明（1900—1993 年）也为战后日本和美国制造业的质量管理做出了重要贡献。他与菲利普·克罗斯比（1926—2001 年）并列为全面质量管理（TQM）之父，并制定了 14 条改进原则。他的工作强项在于拥有渊博的知识体系。他强调，如果真的想在混乱的现实世界中取得进步，需要考虑 4 个宽泛的领域：

- 对于系统的体认。
- 理解与变异相关的知识。

- theory of knowledge
- understanding of psychology.

Crosby, by contrast, in a forerunner of the Six Sigma Approach (see Chapter 4), focused his attention on what he termed the four absolutes of quality. For Crosby, quality is defined as conformance to requirements, not 'goodness' or 'elegance'; the system for causing quality is prevention, not appraisal; the performance standard must be zero defects, not 'that's good enough' and the measurement of quality is the price of nonconformance, not indices.

Finally, *Kaoru Ishikawa* (1915–1989) was a Japanese professor and innovator within the field of quality management and is known for a technique of causal analysis known as the fishbone or Ishikawa diagram (see Chapter 7). Ishikawa led much of the early thinking around quality control and was responsible for the concept of the 'quality circle', where groups of workers involved in similar tasks voluntarily come together regularly to engage in mutual problem definition and problem solving. Still in use today, the approach has led to the widespread adoption of many other participatory management practices.

From higher quality to better value

In recent years, there has been a shift in 'quality thinking' to the related concept of value. Value can be thought of as simply the quality of something divided by its cost. To increase value one either increases the quality or decreases cost, preferably both. However, a more sophisticated view on value, in relation to health, was introduced in 2006 by Michael Porter and Elizabeth Teisbergin their book *Redefining Health Care* (2006).

Porter and Teisberg argued that efforts to reform health care had been hampered by a lack of clarity about goals and that focusing too narrowly on individual dimensions of quality misses the point. In healthcare, the overarching goal must be about improving value for patients. Value in this instance is defined as the health outcomes that matter to patients, relative to the cost of achieving them. Improving value requires either improving outcomes without raising costs or lowering costs without compromising outcomes, or both.

- 理论知识。

- 对心理学的理解。

相反，克罗斯比是六西格玛方法的先驱（见第 4 章），他把注意力集中在四个质量绝对论上。克罗斯比将质量定义为符合要求，而不是良善或优雅；质量的产生是为预防，而不是评价；性能标准必须是零缺陷，而不是足够好；质量测量的依据是不合格的代价，而不是指标。

石川馨（1915–1989 年）是日本质量管理领域的教授和创新者，以因果分析技术而闻名。他发明了鱼骨图，也称为石川图（请参见第 7 章）。石川馨创造了许多有关质量控制的早期理论，并提出了"质量圈"的概念，即参与类似任务的工人定期自愿聚集在一起，共同定义和解决问题，同许多其他参与性的管理实践一样，至今仍被广泛采用。

从高质量到高价值

近年来，质量思维向相关价值观转变。价值可以看作由成本除以某事物质量的模拟。为了增加价值，提高质量或降低成本，最好两者兼而有之。然而，迈克尔·波特和伊丽莎白·泰斯伯格在 2006 年的《重新定义医疗保健》一书中介绍了一种更为复杂的价值观，即与健康有关的价值观。

波特和泰斯伯格认为，改革医疗保健的努力受到目标不明确的阻碍，过于狭隘地关注质量是没有意义的。在医疗保健领域，首要目标是提高患者的医疗价值。在这种情况下，价值被定义为患者的健康。相对于实现这些目标，提高价值要么在不增加成本的情况下改善疗效，要么在不损害结果的情况下降低成本，或者两者兼而有之。

Muir Gray (2015) suggests that a 'value-based' approach to providing services has three important elements:

- Allocative value: allocate resources to different groupsequitably and in a way that maximises value for the whole population.
- Technical value: improve the quality and safety of health-care to increase the value derived from resources allocated to particular services.
- Personalised value: base decisions on the best currentevidence, careful assessment of an individual's clinical condition and an individual's values.

This concept is explored further in Chapter 14 in relation to sustainable approaches expand how value in healthcare can be conceived to include the measurement of health outcomes against environmental, social and financial impacts.

A related concept is that of the Institute of Healthcare Improvement's Triple Aim (2007), a framework that describes an approach to optimising health system performance, applying integrated approaches to simultaneously improve care, improve population health and reduce costs per capita. This approach goes one step further than the detail of Porter's values-based healthcare model and proposes that a population approach and coproduction with stakeholders are essential to create value. The system of healthcare is considered in the round, describing the entire network of prevention, health and social care and focusing on the need and healthcare demand of entire populations. The goal of this coordinated collaboration is then to achieve an optimal outcome in terms of quality, health and costs; the triple aim. See Figure 1.2.

Conclusion

From improving patient safety, to ensuring high-quality care, to value-based approaches and realising the triple aim, there has been a growing sense that the successful health and healthcare systems of the future will be those that can simultaneously deliver excellent quality of care, at optimised costs, while improving the health of the populations that they serve. But to bring about these changes requires the skills, tools and mindsets of quality improvement which the remainder of our book will now go on to describe.

缪尔·格雷于 2015 年提出，提供基于价值的服务具有 3 个重要的要素：

- 分配价值：公平地将资源分配给不同的群体，且分配资源最大化。
- 技术价值：改进医疗保健的质量和安全性，提高将资源分配给特定服务的能力。
- 个性化价值：根据当前的最佳证据做出决定，仔细评估个人的临床状况和个人价值观。

第 14 章进一步探讨了"可持续方法"这一概念，增加了如何构想医疗保健价值，以对环境、社会和财政影响健康状况的评估。

一个相关概念是医疗保健改进研究所提出的三重目标（2007 年），该框架描述了优化医疗系统绩效的方法，采用综合方法改善护理效果及人口健康并降低人均成本。所提出的人口方法比波特基于价值观的医疗模式更进一步，它认为，与利益相关者的合作对创造价值至关重要。全面考虑医疗保健体系，描述了预防、保健和社会护理网络，重点关注全体国民的医疗保健需求。协调协作的目标是在质量、健康和成本方面取得最佳结果，即三重目标。参见图 1.2。

结论

随着改善患者安全、确保高质量护理、以价值为基础的方法和三重目标的提出，人们越来越意识到，未来成功的健康和保健系统将是以较低成本提供优质护理服务的系统，同时能够改善人口健康。但要实现这些变革，需要技能、工具和质量改进的思维方式，本书的其余部分将继续讨论。

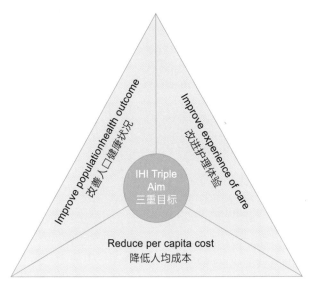

Figure 1.2 The triple aim of healthcare improvement. Source: Berwick et al. (2008).

图1.2 医疗保健改进的三重目标。资料来源：贝里克等（2008年）

References

参考文献

Berwick DM, Nolan TW and Whittington J. (2008) The triple aim: care, health, and cost. *Health Affairs,* 27 (3), 759-769.

Committee on Quality of Health Care in America, Institute of Medicine (2001) *Crossing the Quality Chasm: A New Health System for the 21st Century,* Washington, DC, National Academy Press.

Donabedian A. (1966) Evaluating the quality of medical care. *Milbank Memorial Fund Quarterly* 44 (3) (suppl), 166–206.Reprinted (2005) in Milbank Quarterly 83 (4), 691-729.

Gray M. (2015) A culture of stewardship. The responsibility of NHS leaders to deliver better value healthcare. Academy of Medical Royal Colleges and The NHS Confederation. Available at: https://www.nhsconfed.org/resources/2015/09/a-culture-of-stewardship-the-responsibility-of-nhs-leaders-to-deliver-better-value-healthcare (accessed 19 January 2019).

Institute of Healthcare Improvement (2007) Triple Aim Initiative. Available at: http://www.ihi.org/Engage/Initiatives/TripleAim/ Pages/default.aspx (accessed 4 February 2019).

Kohn LT, Corrigan JM and Donaldson MS (Institute of Medicine) (2000) *To Err is Human: Building a Safer Health System,* Washington, DC, National Academy Press.

NHS England (2016) A shared commitment to quality. Available at: https://www.england.nhs.uk/wp‑content/uploads/2016/12/ nqb-shared-commitment-frmwrk.pdf (accessed 19 January 2019).

Porter ME and Teisberg EO. (2006) *Redefining Health Care: Creating Value-Based Competition on Results,* Boston, MA, Harvard Business School Press.

WHO (2016). What is Quality of Care and why is it important? Maternal, newborn, child and adolescent health. Available at: https://www.who.int/maternal_child_adolescent/topics/ quality-of-care/definition/en/ (accessed 19 January 2019).

Further reading and resources
深度阅读与相关资源

Dale BG, van der Wiele T and Bamford D. (2016) *Managing Quality: An Essential Guide and Resource Gateway,* 6 edn, Oxford, John Wiley & Sons.

Institute of Healthcare Improvement Open School. Available at: www.ihi.org/education/IHIOpenSchool/Courses/Pages/qi102.aspx (accessed 19 January 2019).

NHS Institute for Innovation and Improvement. Quality Improvement: Theory and Practice in Healthcare. Available at: https://qi.elft.nhs.uk/wp-content/uploads/2014/04/quality_improvement-theory_and_practice_in_healthcare1.pdf (accessed 19 January 2019).

第 2 章 | 质量改进

Cat Chatfield

Quality Improvement Editor, The BMJ (British Medical Journal), London, UK

OVERVIEW
概述

- Quality improvement (QI) uses an understanding of our complex healthcare environment and applies a systematic approach to designing, testing and implementing changes using real-time measurement in order to improve the quality of patient care.
  质量改进（QI）利用我们对复杂医疗环境的了解，采用系统的方法，通过实时测量来设计、测试和实施变更，以提高患者护理的质量。

- Much of the history of QI is rooted in the manufacturing industry and a relentless focus on production quality control and organisational change.
  QI 的大部分历史都植根于制造业，并密切关注生产质量控制和组织变革。

- The key concepts in QI include establishing an aim, a diagnostic phase understanding the problem, a problem-solving phaseto test out changes, an evaluation phase measuring the response and an iteration phase developing or sustaining any improvement.
  QI 中的关键概念包括确立目标、理解问题的诊断阶段、测试变更问题的解决阶段、测试响应的评估阶段以及开发或维持任何改进的迭代阶段。

- Quality improvement is a broad umbrella term under which many approaches sit. QI includes audit for improvement, is complementary to patient safety activities, but differs from research and improvement science.
  质量改进是一个宽泛的概念，涉及许多方法。QI 包括改进审计，是对患者安全活动的补充，但不同于研究和改进科学。

What is quality improvement?

In its broadest sense, quality improvement (QI) in health-care means improving the quality of care that patients experience; a definition that might include practising evidence-based medicine or auditing how much care is delivered according to gold standard guidance. In practice, though, QI often describes a specific approach to improving care. The most well-known definition is probably that of Batalden and Davidoff (2007) who describe QI as:

什么是质量改进

从最广泛的意义上讲，医疗质量改进（QI）意味着提高患者的护理质量。该定义可能包括实践循证医学或根据指南金标准提供护理。但是，QI 在实践中常常被描述为改进护理质量的特定方法。最著名的定义可能是巴塔尔登和大卫杜夫（2007 年）提出的，他们将 QI 描述为：

'The combined and unceasing efforts of everyone-healthcare professionals, patients and their families, researchers, payers, planners and educators-to make the changes that will lead to better patient outcomes (health), better system performance (care) and better professional development (learning).'

This considers what QI might be but lacks detail on how we might undertake it. John Ovretveit (2009) addresses this, defining QI as:

'Better patient experience and outcomes achieved through changing provider behaviour and organisation through using a systematic change method and strategies.'

Fully understanding QI requires us to combine and con-textualise these ideas, which can be done under four headings. First, the desired goal. Second, the process by which change is made. Third, those responsible for ensuring these goals are achieved. Fourth, the context within which improvement must take place. See Box 2.1.

"每个人——医疗专业人员、患者及其家属、研究人员、付款人、规划者和教育工作者——一起不断地努力，做出改变，从而带来更好的疗效（健康）、更好的系统性能（护理）和更好的专业发展（学习）。"

这说明了 QI 是什么，但缺乏行动的详细信息。约翰·奥特维特雷特对此进行了阐述（2009 年），将 QI 定义为：

"通过使用系统化的变革方法和策略，改变医疗机构的行为和组织，以获得更好的患者体验和疗效。"

全面了解 QI 要求我们将这些观点结合起来并加以概括，这可以分为 4 个部分。第一，预期目标；第二，改变的过程；第三，负责实现这些目标的人；第四，必须改进的环境。见框 2.1。

Box 2.1 **What is quality improvement?**
框 2.1　**什么是质量改进**

WHAT (goal): Better patient outcomes and experience
是什么（目标）：更好的医疗结果和体验

+

HOW (process): Systematic methods and behaviour change
怎么做（过程）：系统方法和行为改变

+

WHO (people): Healthcare professionals, patients and families, researchers, organisations, commissioners/payers
谁来做（人员）：医疗专业人员、患者和家属、研究人员、组织、专员 / 付款人

+

WHERE (context): In complex health and social systems
在哪里（环境）：在复杂的医疗和社会系统中

Historical context

Epidemiological approaches – dating back to John Snow's identification of a water-pump as the source of a cholera outbreak in London in 1854 – evolved in the twentieth century into clinical epidemiology and the evidence-based medicine movement (Parry 2014). The paradigm of evidence-based medicine (EBM) still underpins much of medical culture.

EBM focuses on a nuanced understanding of research evidence – generated through studies of populations – and then applying this evidence to the care of individual patients. This is a highly effective way of determining what care we should be delivering. But by itself, EBM provides only limited information about how research knowledge should best enter into practice, who should undertake this knowledge transfer and how it can be reliably delivered in a way that improves outcomes for individual patients.

Driven in part by evidence that not all patients were receiving recommended care (McGlynn et al., 2003), and by an increased awareness of the harms caused by healthcare, QI has over the last few decades sought to address these questions by learning from sectors where there has been a relentless focus on quality control and organisational change in implementing and sustaining improvement. These industries have been as diverse as car manufacturing (Deming, Toyota and Lean), management consultancy (the Juran triangle) and telephone engineering (Shewart) with a common grounding in ideas of production, purchase and delivery.

QI challenges us to see outcomes for patients as things that are both produced (based on standards of care defined by evidence-based medicine) and purchased (either by patients or others payers) and so demand a form of thinking aligned not only with epidemiology and EBM, but also with the intricacies of modern manufacturing and service delivery. In this, QI remains nascent and evolving, not least in its ongoing engagement with the ways in which healthcare systems are unique and where (and how) manufacturing paradigms, while useful, fall short of capturing their complexity.

历史背景

流行病学方法可以追溯到 1854 年约翰·斯诺将水泵确定为伦敦霍乱暴发的源头——在 20 世纪演变为临床流行病学和循证医学运动（Parry，2014 年）。循证医学（EBM）范式仍是医学文化的基础。

循证医学致力于人群研究，对产生的研究证据进行深入理解，然后将这些证据应用于个别患者的护理。对于确定我们应该提供什么样的护理，这是一个非常有效的方法。但就其本身而言，循证医学在说明科学研究应该如何更广泛地应用于实践，谁应该进行知识转移，以及如何可靠地传递知识来改善患者健康状况等方面，仅提供了有限的信息。

在一定程度上，有证据表明并非所有患者都得到推荐的治疗（McGlynn 等，2003 年），并且由于人们越来越意识到医疗保健所造成的危害，在过去的几十年里，QI 一直试图通过向那些在实施和持续改进过程中对质量控制和组织变革毫不留情的行业学习，来解决这些问题。这些行业包括汽车制造（戴明、丰田和精益）、管理咨询（朱兰三角）和电话工程（谢沃特），在生产、采购和交付方面有共同的基础。

QI 要求我们将患者的治疗结果视为既是："制造"（基于循证医学定义的护理标准）又是交易（由患者或其他付款人购买），因此不仅需要与流行病学和循证医学保持一致，而且还具有现代制造和服务交付的复杂性。在这一点上，QI 仍然是新概念并需要不断发展，尤其是面对独特的医疗系统，其"制造"模式在哪里（以及如何"制造"）尚未能达到一定的复杂性。

Underpinning concepts

While many thinkers have challenged the idea of thinking about healthcare as producing outcomes as if they were cars on a production line (Batalden, 2018) – particularly the absence of patients as partners in such a mental model – this 'industrial' approach informs many of QI's underpinning ideas. Given that few healthcare professionals are familiar with (say) car manufacturing processes, the following lexicon offers some biological analogues.

Systems

The respiratory and circulatory systems are linked structures and biological processes, each with their own sets of rules, that deliver certain outcomes for our body: oxygenated blood to end-organs, for example. Although we may learn about each individual system, they are all intercon nected and, more importantly, dependent upon each other. When thinking about healthcare and how to do QI, it's important to recognise that the healthcare system is itself a series of interconnected, interdependent processes and pathways. This is particularly important when considering unexpected consequences in different parts of the system: for example, how changing the way patients are discharged from the medical assessment unit in a hospital might impact on the pharmacy, discharge lounge or transport. It's also important for understanding how complex systems may resist change – and how different parts of the systemshave different priorities and approaches.

Processes

Thinking in terms of processes can help us understand the work or actions done within a system by breaking them down into a series of discrete steps, linked in a particular order.

Consider the process of obtaining energy from the food we eat: we put food in our mouth, tear it up with our teeth, release salivary enzymes, swallow the food into our oesophagus, etc. We can view a process in primary care along similar lines: a patient is running out of their medication, submits a repeat prescription request via email, it goes into the reception inbox, an administrator passes it on to a GP for reauthorisation, etc.

基础概念

虽然许多思想家质疑将医疗保健视为与生产线上的汽车一样产生效益的想法（Batalden，2018 年）——尤其在这种疯狂的模式中没有把患者当作合作伙伴——这种工业方法激发出了许多 QI 的基础思想。鉴于很少有医疗专业人员熟悉（比如说）汽车制造过程，下面的概念采用了一些与生物学相关的阐述。

系统

呼吸系统和循环系统相互联系，共同维持生命过程，每个系统都有自己的规则和作用。例如，血液可将氧气送达机体末端。每个系统相互联系、相互依赖。在思考医疗和如何进行 QI 时，必须意识到医疗系统本身就是一系列相互关联、相互依存的过程和路径。在考虑系统不同部分的意外后果时，这一点尤为重要。例如，改变患者出院的方式可能会对药房、病房或交通产生影响。这对于理解复杂的系统如何抵御变革，以及系统各个部分如何设置优先级并处理也很重要。

流程

从流程的角度来思考可以帮助理解系统中所做的工作或行为，方法是将它们分解为一系列离散的步骤，并按特定的顺序联系起来。

考虑从吃的食物中获取能量的流程：把食物放入嘴里，用牙齿撕碎，释放消化酶，把食物咽进食管等。我们可以按照类似的路线看待初级保健流程：患者的药物用完，通过电子邮件再次提交处方申请，管理员进入处方收件箱，将其交给全科医生重新授权等。

Understanding the work we do as a process helps us to see which parts of the system are working well or not so well, how different sections of the system overlap, and where we might change them.

Flow

Once we start seeing healthcare as a system of interconnected processes and pathways, we can think about how patients move through this system: the concept of flow.

Consider symptoms of poor urinary flow: we need to understand where the obstruction is occurring – a urethral stricture or an enlarged prostate, for example. Each have very different treatments. The same applies to our healthcare systems.

Looking at patient flow helps us to identify where bottlenecks occur – those parts of a process that slow down patient flow – or where patients are having to go through 'waste' processes that don't improve their experience or outcomes.

One major challenge for flow is that patients move across the whole system, from home to primary care, out of hours care, secondary care and back again. Making improvement across these boundaries is vitally important when trying to achieve better outcomes.

Variation

Variation describes when processes or outcomes of care differ from what might be recommended. Anyone working in healthcare is familiar with variation: not every hip fracture is the same, not every patient with a hip fracture receives the same treatment.

Warranted or 'good' variation is when clinical care differs from guideline-recommended care for good reasons, such as patient preference, priorities or clinical judgement. A patient with a hip fracture secondary to a bony metastasis may benefit more from radiotherapy or analgesia than a surgical intervention, for example.

By contrast, unwarranted variation describes care that differs from recommended standards for no obviously good reason: a clear target for improving the quality of healthcare.

了解流程中工作有助于了解系统的哪些部分运行良好或运行不正常，系统各个部分如何重叠，以及可以在哪里更改。

"流"（质控流程）

一旦将医疗视为由相互关联的流程和路径组成的系统，我们就可以思考患者如何通过这个系统，这就是"流"。

考虑一下尿流不畅的症状，这需要了解梗阻的发生部位——例如尿道狭窄或前列腺肥大，每个人都有非常不同的治疗方法。这同样适用于医疗体系。

观察"患者流"有助于确定哪里出现了瓶颈：流程中那些减慢"患者流"的部分，或者患者不得不经历那些无法改善其体验或结果的冗余流程。

"流"的一个主要难题是患者从家庭到初级保健、非工时保健、二级保健到再次返回的整个系统。在努力取得更好的结果时，这些跨越边界的改进至关重要。

变异

"变异"描述了护理的流程或结果可能与指南建议的不同。任何从事医疗保健工作的人都熟悉这种变异：并非每个髋部骨折的情形都是相同的，也并非每个髋部骨折患者都接受相同的治疗。

有保证或良好变异是指临床护理出于好的出发点（如患者偏好、优先级或临床判断）而采取不同于指南建议的护理。例如，继发于骨转移的髋部骨折患者可能更受益于放射治疗或镇痛，而不是外科手术。

相比之下，不合理的变异描述的是，在不能明显提高医疗质量的情况下，采用不同于推荐标准的护理。

Common cause and special variation are terms used in statistical process control when interpreting Shewart or Control charts (see Chapter 9).

共因变异和特殊变异是在解释 Shewart 或控制图表统计流程控制时使用的术语（参见第 9 章）。

The quality improvement process

QI can be presented as a specific approach or method, such as the Model for Improvement (Langley et al. 1996), Lean or Design Thinking, but can also incorporate different approaches used in systematic ways. For example, a project aiming to improve how patients receive blood test results may use a Design Thinking approach to develop and iterate a patient-facing online result portal, but Lean workshops to identify improvements in the way the laboratory handles samples. Current evidence does not suggest the superiority of one approach or method over another – but this is partly because the evidence base for QI overall is limited (Dixon - Woods, 2019).

The core features of most QI approaches include a diagnostic phase; spending time understanding the problem through various methods and tools. This is followed by a problem-solving phase, which usually involves testing ideas of change; for example, through prototypes, ideation or through implementing small changes in processes. QI must then proceed to an evaluation phase, where the ideas or changes are assessed against the aims and the theory of change. Finally, it should include an iteration phase, where changes are revised and repeated (Figure 2.1).

质量改进流程

QI 可以用具体的方式或方法来表示，例如改进模型（Langley 等，1996 年）、精益或设计思维，但也可以在系统中将各种方法结合起来使用。例如，旨在影响患者如何接受血液检测结果的项目，可以使用设计思维方法来开发和迭代面向患者的在线显示结果的网站，精益研讨会可改进实验室处理样本的方式。目前的证据并不能表明一种方式或方法比另一种优越，但这个结论部分是因为 QI 整体的证据基础有限（Dixon-Woods，2019年）。

大多数 QI 方法的核心特征包括在诊断阶段花时间通过各种方法和工具来理解问题；接下来是问题解决阶段，通常通过原型、构思或实施过程中的小变化来测试改进方案。然后进入评估阶段，根据目标和变革理论对想法或改进进行评估。最后，还应该包括修改和重复变更的迭代阶段（图 2.1）。

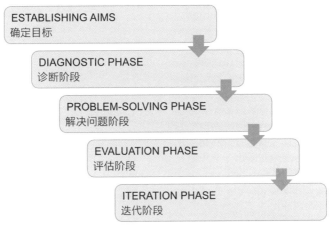

All informed by a THEORY OF CHANGE and underpinned by DATA
所有内容均以"变革理论"为依据，并以"数据"为基础

Figure 2.1 The quality improvement process.

图 2.1   质量改进流程

In order to move through these phases, two other core features of QI are required: a theory of change and data. A theory of change is similar to a scientific hypothesis: it sets out our thinking about how and why our proposed change idea might move us closer to achieving our desired improvement (Moonesinghe and Peden, 2017).

In some ways, this maps a process close to clinical problem-solving. In a clinician's examination of a wheezy child, for example:

- I need to improve their current symptoms and make a diagnosis (AIM).
- But … I'm not sure whether this wheezy child has a viral illness or undiagnosed asthma (Problem requiring DIAGNOSIS).
- So … if I measure their peak expiratory flow rate during this episode of wheeze then I'll have a baseline measure (Gathering DATA).
- If … I initiate inhaled corticosteroid therapy that should improve their symptoms (PROBLEM SOLVING according to THEORY OF CHANGE).
- Then … I can review them again to see if their peak flow has improved and assess them for the results of a trial of treatment (EVALUATION through DATA).
- If … they haven't improved, then I can change their treatment or reconsider my diagnosis (ITERATION).
- Therefore … I have a plan for treating their wheeze and also making it more likely I can make a diagnosis (AIM).

We are unlikely to initiate any treatment for a patient without having some way of assessing its impact. Similarly, QI must include meaningful measures of whether change has improved outcomes and experience of care for patients.

These measures can be qualitative or quantitative – multiple categories of evidence are required to engage with any complex system. Just as asking patients about their experience of taking medication can help identify side-effects and how likely they are to sustain treatment, asking staff about their experience of training to use a new pathology results system helps to build up a picture of factors which made implementing change easier or more difficult.

为了跨越这些阶段，需要 QI 的其他 2 个核心功能：变革理论和数据。变革理论类似科学假设：它阐明了对变革理论的思考，即如何以及为什么能够使实现期望的改进（Moonesinghe 和 Peden，2017 年）。

在某些方面，这体现了类似临床问题的解决流程。例如，临床医生给 1 个喘息儿童做检查：

- 我需要改善他目前的症状并做出诊断（目标）。
- 但是我不确定这个喘息的孩子是病毒性疾病还是未确诊的哮喘（问题需要诊断）。
- 所以如果我在喘息发作期间测量他的呼气流量峰值，那么我将得到 1 个基线测量值（收集数据）。
- 如果我给予吸入糖皮质激素治疗，应该可以改善症状（根据变革理论解决问题）。
- 然后我可以再次检查，看看他的流量峰值是否有所改善，并评估治疗试验结果（通过数据评估）。
- 如果他没有改善，那么我可以改变治疗方案或重新考虑诊断（迭代）。
- 因此我制订 1 个计划来治疗他的喘息，并让我更有可能做出诊断（目标）。

如果没有某种评估其影响的方法，我们不太可能对患者进行任何治疗。同样，QI 必须包括有意义的衡量标准，以测量变更是否改善了患者的疗效和体验。

这些衡量标准可以是定性的，也可以是定量的——任何复杂的系统都需要多种类型的证据。正如询问患者服用药物史有助于确定副作用以及维持治疗的可能性，询问员工新型病理系统培训体验有助于了解实施变更更容易或更困难的因素。

Measurement in QI is also important for assessing a theory of change versus the reality of what is observed and experienced. For this reason, the evaluation phase of QI should not only focus on whether change generated improvement but how and why this happened.

Finally, QI data should always be measured over time. This enables the effect of changes to be seen on systems, processes and outcomes – and is vital for assessing both the sustainability of improvement, and whether it may simply be attributable to normal variation in outcomes. There is often confusion over whether clinical audit is a QI approach. It can be; but only when used to repeatedly cycle through a process that continuously improves the quality of care (Box 2.2).

What quality improvement is not

Research

Research is a systematic investigation designed to develop or contribute to generalisable knowledge and proof of effectiveness of what is the right thing to do in the care of our patients. QI provides the means to translate the best evidence into practice adapting for local context, culture and conditions.

QI 的测量对于评估变革理论与观察和体验事实的真实性也很重要。因此，QI 的评估阶段不仅应关注变更是否产生了改进，还应关注这种变更发生的方式和原因。

最后，应长期测量 QI 数据。这可以看到变更对系统、流程和结果的影响，对于评估改进的可持续性以及判断结果的正常变化都至关重要。关于临床审计是否为一种 QI 方法，这一点常常令人困惑。它可以是，但仅用于持续提高护理质量这一循环流程（框 2.2）。

质量改进不是什么

研究

研究属于系统性调查，旨在发展或促进知识的推广和对患者正确治疗有效性的证明。QI 提供了将最佳证据转化为适合当地情况、文化和条件的实践方法。

Box 2.2 **Quality improvement and clinical audit.**
框 2.2　**质量改进和临床审计**

Clinical audit is a quality improvement process that seeks to improve patient care and outcomes through the systematic review of care against explicit criteria and the implementation of change (Flottorp et al., 2010). Potential confusion over clinical audit as a QI approach has arisen from its dual role as a quality assurance process and as an improvement process.

临床审计是一个质量改进过程，旨在通过根据标准和变更实施情况对护理进行系统审查来改善患者的护理效果（Flottorp 等，2010 年）。临床审计作为 QI 方法可能产生的混淆源于其作为质量保证过程和改进流程的双重作用。

By focusing on quality assurance, small adjustments in practice are made to conform to standards rather than taking every opportunity to improve care. By shifting from an emphasis on one-off time aggregated data collections, to repeated cycles with time ordered data to measure and evaluate the impact of a change, audit becomes a useful tool for continuous improvement.

注重质量保证，在实践中进行小的调整以符合标准，而不是抓住每个机会来改善护理效果。数据从一次性的时间汇总收集改至持续收集按时间排序的周期性数据来测量和评估变更的影响，审计会成为持续改进的有用工具。

Improvement science

The term 'improvement science' is used to refer to the scientific study of the methods and factors that facilitate how quality improvement is done, drawing on interdisciplinary research methods from across clinical and social sciences. Improvement science aims to generate systematic generalisable knowledge about how to improve the quality and safety of healthcare. It differs from clinical science research, which aims at generalisable knowledge about what interventions, approaches or treatments make highquality care.

Patient safety

Patient safety and QI activities complement each other. Patient safety initiatives aim to identify and then prevent or mitigate errors or adverse outcomes for patients as a result of care. QI aims to ensure all patients receive appropriate care in a timely fashion according to their needs. QI activities aim to 'raise the ceiling' in healthcare, while patient safety activities aim to 'raise the floor' (Stevens et al., 2005). See Figure 2.2.

改进科学

"改进科学"一词是指利用临床和社会科学的跨学科研究方法，对促进质量改进的方法和因素进行科学研究。"改进科学"的目的是产生关于如何系统性提高医疗质量和安全性的一般性知识。它与临床科学研究不同，后者的目的是提供用于高质量护理的干预措施、方法或疗法的一般性知识。

患者安全

患者安全与 QI 活动相辅相成。提出患者安全倡议旨在识别并预防或减轻因护理而给患者带来的伤害或不良后果。QI 的目标是确保所有患者根据他们的需要及时得到适当的护理。QI 活动旨在"提高医疗的上限"，而患者安全活动旨在"提高下限"（Stevens 等，2005 年）。见图 2.2。

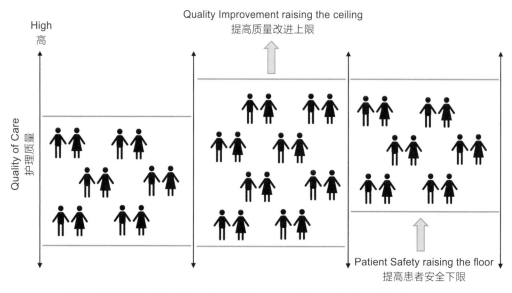

Figure 2.2 Raising the ceiling. Source: Stevens et al. (2005). Adapted with permission.

图 2.2 提高上限。资料来源：史蒂文斯等（2005 年），经允许改编

Conclusion

QI is not a panacea which will solve all the problems of delivering high-quality healthcare in partnership with patients in a complex environment. It does provide a process and a set of tools and methods which can help us move systematically towards thinking about creating and improving better quality care.

结论

QI 不能解决在复杂环境中为患者提供高质量医疗服务所遇到的所有问题。但它确实提供了流程、工具和方法，可以帮助我们系统地朝着思考如何建立和改进护理质量的方向迈进。

References
参考文献

Batalden PB and Davidoff F. (2007) What is 'quality improvement' and how can it transform healthcare? *Quality and Safety in Health Care* 16 (1), 2-3.

Batalden P. (2018) Getting more health from healthcare: quality improvement must acknowledge patient coproduction – an essay by Paul Batalden. *British Medical Journal* 362, k3617.

Dixon-Woods M. (2019) Harveian Oration 2018: Improving quality and safety in healthcare. *Clinical Medicine*, 19 (1), 47-56.

Flottorp S, Jamtvedt G, Gibis B et al. (2010) *Using Audit and Feedback to Health Professionals to Improve the Quality and Safety of Health care*. World Health Organization Health Evidence Network, Geneva, WHO.

Langley GL, Nolan KM, Nolan TW et al. (1996) *The Improvement Guide: A Practical Approach to Enhancing Organizational Performance*, San Francisco, Jossey-Bass.

McGlynn EA, Asch SM, Adams J et al. (2003) The quality of health care delivered to adults in the United States. *New England Journal of Medicine*, 348, 2635-2645.

Moonesinghe SR and Peden CJ. (2017) Theory and context: putting the science into improvement. *British Journal of Anaesthesia*, 118 (4), 482-484.

Øvretveit J. (2009) *Does Improving Quality Save Money? A Review of the Evidence of which Improvements to Quality Reduce Costs to Health Service Providers,* London, Health Foundation.

Parry JA. (2014) Brief history of quality improvement. *Journal of Oncology Practice*, 10 (3), 196-199.

Stevens P, Matlow A and Laxer R. (2005) Building from the blueprint for patient safety at the hospital for sick children. *Healthcare Quarterly*, 8 (Sp), 132-139.

Further reading and resources
深度阅读与相关资源

Jones B, Vaux E and Olsson-Brown A. (2019) How to get started in quality improvement. *British Medical Journal* 364, k5408.

The Health Foundation (2012) Overcoming challenges to improving quality. Available at: www.health.org.uk/publication/ overcoming-challenges-improving-quality (accessed 15 May 2019).

The Health Foundation (2013) Quality improvement made simple. Available at: www.health.org.uk/publication/qualityimprovement-made-simple (accessed 15 May 2019).

Chapter 3

Quality Improvement and the Healthcare Professional

质量改进与医疗专业人员

Tricia Woodhead

Health Foundation and Institute of Healthcare Improvement Quality Improvement Fellow, London, UK

OVERVIEW
概述

- Optimal care arises from the application of the knowledge, skills and behaviours of excellent clinicians, managers and support staff working with patients, families and carers.

  最佳护理需要优秀临床医生、管理人员和支持人员投入知识、技能和行动，他们与患者、家属和护理人员合作。

- Quality improvement approaches support and enable healthcare professionals to meet their duty to make the care of the patient their first concern, to design and deliver safe and high-quality services and work in, and lead, high-performing teams.

  质量改进方法为医疗保健专业人员提供支持并使其履行职责，将患者的护理作为首要关注点，设计和提供安全和高质量的服务，并让团队工作更高效。

- All healthcare professionals should be able to participate in, and develop the competences and confidence to apply, quality improvement methods.

  所有医疗专业人员都应该使用质量改进方法，并培养应用质量改进方法的能力和信心。

- Ideally, all healthcare professionals will also work in a supportive organisational environment of continuous learning.

  理想情况下，所有医疗专业人员也将在能持续学习的支持性组织环境中工作。

- Quality improvement activities enable team members to work and learn together to develop skills in managing complexity and leading change and understand the impact of human factors and how to involve patients throughout the improvement process.

  质量改进活动需团队成员一起工作和学习，以开发管理复杂性和引领变更的技能，并了解人为因素的影响以及如何使患者参与整个改进过程。

Improvement in healthcare

Healthcare professionals practise in complex systems where learning and continuous improvement should be supported by everyone. All healthcare professionals are expected to have and maintain the necessary knowledge, personal skills and behaviours to ensure patients are always cared for effectively and compassionately. These expectations are described in codes of practice and they have been adapted to meet new and changing contexts as well as developments

医疗改进

医疗保健专业人员在复杂的系统中行医，每个人都应不断学习和持续改进。医疗专业人员应有必要的知识、个人技能和行动，以确保始终有效而富有同情心地照顾患者。实践准则描述了这些期望，并调整以适应新的环境以及医学的发展。框 3.1 针对英国的医生和护士提供了 2 个现行职业实践守则的摘

Box 3.1 **Professional codes of practice.**
框 3.1　职业行医守则

General Medical Council UK, Good Medical Practice (2018)
英国医学总会，优质临床医疗指南（2018 年）

- Make the care of the patient your first concern.
  把护理患者作为第一要务。

- Be competent and keep your practice up to date.
  有能力，并不断更新技能。

- Take prompt action if you think patient care has been compromised.
  如果你认为患者护理受到影响，请立即采取行动。

- Establish and maintain good partnerships with patients.
  与患者建立并保持良好的合作关系。

- Maintain trust in you and in the profession.
  对自己和这个职业保持信任。

Source: www.gmc-uk.org/ethical - guidance/ethical-guidance-fordoctors/good-medical-practice.
来源：www.gmc-uk.org/ethical-guidance/ethical-guidance-fordoctors/good-medical-practice。

Nursing and Midwifery Council UK, Professional Practice Standards (2018)
英国护理和助产协会，职业临床护理指南（2018 年）

- Prioritise people.
  以人为本。

- Practise effectively.
  有效护理。

- Preserve safety.
  保证安全。

- Provide professionalism and trust.
  专业尽责。

Source: www.nmc.org.uk/standards/code.
来源：www.nmc.org.uk/standards/code。

---

in medical science. Box 3.1 provides summary examples of two current professional codes of practice: for doctors and nurses in the UK.

While medical advances have created tremendous opportunity for improved treatment and survival, they have also created new challenges for professionals. Better outcomes for patients come from constant professional development, excellent individual performance and behaviour but also require improved 'whole system' performance. Batalden and Davidoff (2007) describe the necessary knowledge systems involved in healthcare improvement as being: scientific knowledge, contextual awareness, performance measurement, plans for change and execution of those planned changes.

要示例。

医学的进步为改进治疗方案和提高寿命创造了巨大的机会，同时也给专业人员带来了新的挑战。患者更好的疗效来自专业不断的发展、出色的个人表现和行为，但也需要改进整个系统的性能。巴塔尔登和大卫杜夫（2007 年）描述了医疗改进所涉及的必要知识体系：科学知识、背景意识、绩效测量、变革计划和计划的执行。他们观察到："每个从事医疗工作的人每天上班时都有 2 份工作——本职工作和改进工作。"

They observe that: 'everyone in healthcare really has two jobs when they come to work every day: to do their work and to improve it.'

Professional codes of practice for medical, nursing and allied healthcare professionals require individuals to maintain their skills, take prompt action if there are safety concerns and work in teams, and with patients, to maintain trust. However, healthcare professionals all work within healthcare organisations and systems alongside managers and other staff who may also have project management skills and operational knowledge that are needed to make change that is an improvement. All staff have a role to play in ensuring patients are always safe and receive high-quality care (see Figure 3.1).

Quality is everyone's responsibility

Increasingly, over the last 20 years, it has been recognised that healthcare organisations require a deliberate, systemwide, approach to quality and safety to enable a culture of continuous improvement with staff encouraged to participate at all levels and stages of their career. The consequences of failure to do this were clearly described in the UK by Don Berwick (2013) in his learning from the 'Francis Report' (Report of the Mid-Staffordshire NHS Foundation Trust public inquiry) and are summarised in Box

医疗、护理和相关医疗专业人员的职业实践守则要求个人始终掌握技能,在存在安全问题时立即采取行动,并与患者合作,以保持信任。然而,医疗专业人员都在医疗组织和系统内,与管理人员和其他工作人员一起工作,他们可能还具有项目管理技能和实践知识,这些技能和知识是改进所必需的。所有员工都应在确保患者始终安全和接受高质量护理方面发挥作用(见图 3.1)。

保证质量是每个人的责任

过去 20 年,人们逐渐意识到,医疗机构需要一种审慎的、全系统的质量和安全方法,以塑造持续改进的文化,鼓励员工参与其职业生涯的各个阶段和层面。唐·伯威克(2013年)在英国从"弗朗西斯报告"(斯塔福德郡 NHS 基金会信托基金公开查询的报告)中清楚地描述了未能做到这点的后果,并在框 3.2 中进行了总结。国际上已经在医疗系统中

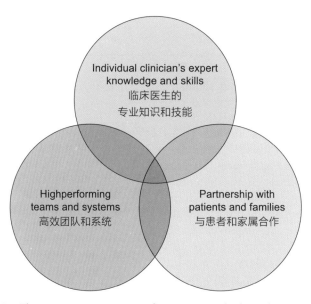

Figure 3.1 The components necessary for continuous high-quality patient care.

图 3.1 持续高质量患者护理的构成

3.2. New and more extensive efforts have been made across healthcare systems internationally to ensure that the quality and safety of patient care is both an individual's responsibility but is always within and supported by a whole system 'learning environment' that creates the right environment to improve. You can read more on cultures of improvement in Chapter 13.

做出了新的、更多的努力，以确保患者护理的质量和安全，这既是每个医护人员的责任，又需要整个系统始终处于"学习环境"，才能创造适当的环境来改进。你可以在第 13 章阅读更多关于改进文化的内容。

Box 3.2 **A promise to learn – a commitment to act.**

框 3.2　**学习的承诺——行动的承诺**

In 2013, an independent group of experts in quality improvement, patient safety and organisational and systems theories, led by Don Berwick, President Emeritus of the Institute of Healthcare Improvement, was commissioned to review issues that compromise patient safety in England's National Health Service (NHS). The report followed events that led to serious lapses in patient care at Mid Staffordshire Hospitals and made a number of recommendations for the NHS to address both in relation to unsafe care at Mid Staffordshire and other patient safety issues that could lead to harm elsewhere in the NHS.

2013 年，一个独立的质量改进、患者安全以及组织和系统理论专家组，由医疗保健改善研究所名誉院长唐·伯威克领导，受委托审查英格兰的英国国家医疗服务体系（NHS）中危及患者安全的问题。该报告跟踪了中斯塔福德郡医院患者护理严重失误事件，并为 NHS 提出了一些建议，以解决与中斯塔福德郡不安全护理有关的问题，防止伤害 NHS 其他地方的患者。

The recommendations to improve systems, safety and culture in the English NHS are broadly applicable to other healthcare institutions and settings.

NHS 关于改进系统、安全和文化的建议广泛适用于其他地区的医疗机构。

A Promise to Learn – a Commitment to Act (2013) exhorts all organisations providing healthcare to:

《学习的承诺——行动的承诺》（2013 年）鼓励所有提供医疗保健服务的组织：

- Place the quality of patient care, especially patient safety, above all other aims.

  将患者护理的质量，特别是患者安全放在所有其他目标之上。

- Engage, empower and hear patients and carers at all times.

  随时参与、授权和听取患者和护理人员的意见。

- Foster whole-heartedly the growth and development of all staff, including their ability, and support to improve the processes in which they work.

  全心全意地促进所有医护人员的成长和发展，包括提高他们的能力，以及支持其改进工作的流程。

- Embrace transparency unequivocally and everywhere, in the service of accountability, trust and the growth of knowledge.

  对于问责制、信任和知识增长型的服务体系，应保证透明。

Quality improvement – a core clinical skill

Improving healthcare should be the work of everyone, as individuals and as a wider team. As Batalden and Davidoff (2007) state:

'healthcare will not realise its full potential unless change making becomes an intrinsic part of everyone's job, every day, in all parts of the system.'

There is no doubt that with increasingly rapid developments in medical science and models of delivery, systems of healthcare provision have become vastly more complex – as has ensuring their reliability. To date, professional education and training has focused on specific clinical knowledge and skills, rather than an ability to work on the system in which it is practised. To equip professionals to respond to such challenges requires the embedding of improvement methodology as a core competence in practice for all healthcare professionals (Figure 3.2).

Key requirements identified to be able to achieve this include strategic and supporting infrastructure at multiple levels – including within hospital trusts and boards, education, training and continued professional development of all healthcare professionals and supporting resources including provision of time within a job plan to invest in quality improvement activities and nurturing networks (Health Foundation 2012; Academy of Medical Royal Colleges 2016).

质量改进——核心临床技能

改善医疗保健服务应该是个体和团队中每个人的工作。正如巴塔尔登和大卫杜夫（2007 年）所说：

"除非变革成为系统各个部分每天工作中必不可少的一部分，否则医疗将无法发挥其全部潜力。"

毫无疑问，随着医学和交付模式的快速发展，为了确保其可靠性，医疗保健系统变得更加复杂。迄今为止，专业教育和培训侧重于具体的临床知识和技能，而不是实践的能力。为了让专业人员应对这些挑战，需要将实践改进方法作为所有医疗专业人员实践中的核心能力（图 3.2）。

能够实现这一目标的关键要求包括多个层面——医院信托机构和董事会内部的战略和基础设施支持，教育、培训和所有医疗专业人员持续的技能学习以及配套支持性资源，包括在工作计划中腾出时间以投资质量改进活动和培育网络（健康基金会，2012 年；皇家医学院，2016 年）。

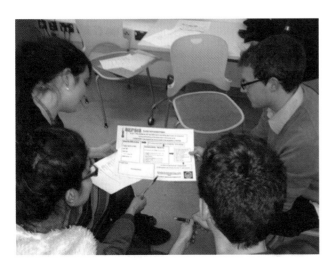

Figure 3.2 Improvement – a core clinical competence for all healthcare professionals.
图 3.2 改进——所有医疗专业人员的核心临床能力

Improving care together

Technical advances and rapidly advancing medical knowledge have accelerated the need for change in healthcare in recent decades. In addition, long-term conditions have increased in prevalence across all countries creating new challenges for health and social care systems and professionals. When ill health is more likely to be a long-term condition than a single event, the need for excellent communication over time with all those involved becomes crucial. Working closely with patients and their families as partners in co-producing the best outcome is increasingly important for effective care but also to ensure the most efficient use of resources.

Quality improvement enables healthcare professionals to successfully improve care through the deployment of methods specifically developed to enable change in complex environments. Using proven quality improvement approaches ensures that all healthcare staff share and understand a common language when discussing improvement. It also allows patients, families and the public to participate and share that language and the data and contribute ideas for change that matter to them. This in turn enables system-wide collaboration, building will, working with patients, coaching teams, improving data collection and its use, integrating pathways for patients and putting local ideas for improvement into practice and then sharing these more widely. A recent example is the National Maternal and Neonatal Health Safety Collaborative in England (NHS Improvement, 2019). The principles of 'all share all learn' and that quality improvement is a team activity are evident in the aims and the design of such collaboratives.

Generic professional capabilities

Quality improvement activities bring members of teams to work and learn together developing transferable skills in managing complexity and leading change. Essential to improvement change is supportive leadership which focuses on valuing the viewpoint, skills and expertise of others, creating networks for connecting and collaboration, and building confidence and trust in each other. Alignment of purpose,

共同改进护理

近几十年，技术进步和医学的迅速发展加速了医疗保健变革的需求。此外，全球各国的慢性患者都在增加，给医疗和社会保健系统及其专业人员带来了新的挑战。当疾病是长期病症而不是单次发病时，随着时间的推移，所有相关人员进行良好沟通变得至关重要。与患者及家人密切合作，对于有效护理以及确保资源的高效利用越来越重要。

质量改进使医疗专业人员能够使用先进方法来成功地改进护理，从而适应复杂的环境。使用经过验证的质量改进方法可确保所有医务人员在讨论改进时分享并理解"同一语言"。它还允许患者、家属和公众参与并共享该"语言"和数据，并为对他们重要的变更提供想法。这反过来又使医护人员愿意与患者合作，并辅助团队，改进数据收集及使用，为患者整合治疗路程径，将当地的改进想法付诸实践，然后更广泛地分享这些想法。最近的一个例子是英国的孕产妇和新生儿健康安全合作组织（英国国家医疗服务体系改进委员会，2019 年）提出"大家共享，大家学习"作为团队质量改进活动的原则，让协作的目标和设计更明确。

通用的专业能力

质量改进活动使团队成员共同努力学习开发、管理复杂的变革和引领变革的可转移技能。改进变革的关键是有领导支持，其重点是重视他人的观点、技能和专业知识，建立连接和协作网络及彼此的信心和信任。在质量改进活动中，一个团体的目标、方法和

methodologies and connectedness across a group of people undertaking a quality improvement activity is just as important as alignment of purpose, methodologies and connectedness in improvement activities undertaken across a system.

In addition, the increased knowledge and application of human factors science has enabled us to build more resilient ways to care for patients (Russ et al., 2013). When we understand why and when humans make an error or a mistake, we can build a better way to do the work to either prevent or to catch that mistake before it causes needless harm. By doing so any improvement change design is strengthened and underpinned by being mindful of human factors at play. One example is the use of data to learn from rather than to be judged by or blamed for. This enables the team to learn and develop as they explore and implement a better way to provide high-quality care.

Conclusion

The Health Foundation's Habits of an Improver (Figure 3.3) describes the key charact-eristics that healthcare improvers should develop and nurture in themselves and others. Co-producing health with colleagues, patients and families has at its core good communication but it also requires active learning, influencing, resilience, creativity and systems thinking. Healthcare professionals seeking to improve their work and the care of their patients can develop and nurture these habits. In addition, increasing evidence shows that front line involvement in change using these approaches provides 'joy in work' (Perlo et al., 2017). The experience that colleagues can gain in taking an idea, testing it out, measuring the impact and then refining and spreading that improvement is empowering and motivating.

Caring for people is both technical and emotional work. Participating in quality improvement work builds an environment that nurtures improved practice through actions, attitudes and behaviours. Quality improvement approaches provide the mechanism by which this aspiration can become a reality.

联结与整个系统改进活动的目的、方法和联结同样重要。

此外，主动获取科学知识并应用能够建立更有弹性的护理患者的方法（Russ 等，2013 年）。理解人类为什么以及何时会犯错误，就可以构建更好的方法来工作，以防止产生或发现错误，从而避免不必要的伤害。这样，通过关注人为因素，可以更好地改进变革。如利用数据来学习，而不是评判或指责。这让团队在探索和实施更好的方法来提供高质量护理的过程中学习和成长。

结论

健康基金会提出的改进者习惯（图 3.3）描述了医疗改进者应具有的需要从自身和他人身上培育和发展的关键特征。与同事、患者和家属共同创造健康关系的核心是良好的沟通，但也需要主动学习，有影响力、适应力、创造力和系统思维。既要参与改进工作，又要照顾患者的医疗专业人员可以培养这些习惯。此外，越来越多的证据表明，使用这些方法参与一线变革可以在工作中找到快乐（Perlo 等，2017 年）。同事在构思、测试、评估后果，然后细化和扩大改进活动后所获得的经验可以鼓舞和激励他人。

护理他人既是技术工作，也是情感工作。参与质量改进工作，将建立一个通过行动、态度和行为来培育改进实践的环境。质量改进方法提供了使这一愿望变为现实的机制。

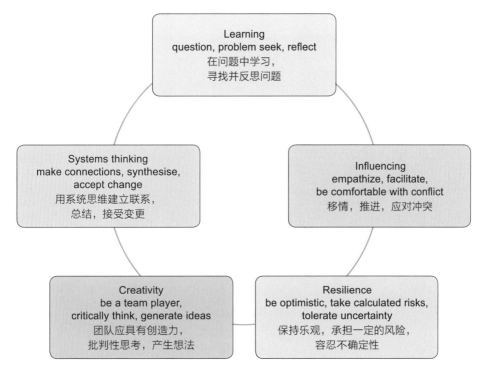

Figure 3.3 Personal and team habits for improvement. Source: Adapted from Lucas and Nacer (2015).

图 3.3　个人和团队的改进习惯。资料来源：改编自卢卡斯和纳赛尔（2015 年）

References
参考文献

Academy of Medical Royal Colleges (2016) *Training for Better Outcomes*, London, Academy of Medical Royal Colleges. Available at: https://www.aomrc.org.uk/wp‑content/uploads/2016/06/ Quality_improvement_key_findings_140316‑2.pdf. (accessed 15 May 2019).

Batalden P and Davidoff F. (2007) What is quality improvement and how can it transform healthcare? *Quality and Safety in Healthcare*, 16, 2-3.

Berwick D. (2013) *A Promise To Learn – A Commitment To Act: Improving The Safety Of Patients In England*. Available at: www.gov. uk/government/publications/berwick‑review‑into‑patient‑safety (accessed 15 May 2019).

Lucas W and Nacer H. (2015) *The Habits of an Improver*, London, The Health Foundation. Available at: www.health.org.uk/ publications/the-habits-of-an-improver (accessed 15 May 2019).

NHS Improvement (2019) *Maternal and Neonatal Health Improvement Collaborative*. Available at: https:// improvement.nhs.uk/resources/maternal-and-neonatal-safety-collaborative/ (accessed 15 May 2019).

Perlo J, Balik B, Swensen S et al. (2017) *IHI Framework for Improving Joy at Work*, Boston, Massachusetts, USA, Institute for Healthcare Improvement. Available at: www.ihi.org/Topics/ Joy-In-Work/Pages/default.aspx (accessed 15 May 2019).

Russ AL, Fairbanks RJ, Karsh B et al. (2013) *The science of human factors: separating fact from fiction. BMJ Quality & Safety*, 22, 802-808.

The Health Foundation (2012) *Quality Improvement Training for Healthcare Professionals*, London, The Health Foundation. Available at: https://www.health.org.uk/publications/qualityimprovement‑training‑for‑healthcare‑professionals (accessed 15 May 2019).

Further reading and resources
深度阅读与相关资源

NHS Scotland. *Quality Improvement Curriculum Framework*. Available at: www.qihub.scot.nhs.uk/media/219075/quality% 20improvement%20curriculum%20framework_03.10.11.pdf (accessed 15 May 2019).

Tweedie J, Harden J and Dacre J. (2018) *Advancing Medical Professionalism*, London, Royal College of Physicians. Available at: https://www.rcplondon.ac.uk/projects/outputs/advancingmedical-professionalism (accessed 15 May 2019).

Karen Evans

Director of Delivery, Alamac Ltd, Northall, UK

OVERVIEW
概述

- Successful healthcare organisations adopt a clear organisational approach to quality improvement, based on specific models.
  成功的医疗机构根据具体模型来制订明确的组织方法进而提高质量。
- Four of the most commonly used models are Lean, the Model for Improvement, Six Sigma and Experience-based Co-design.
  4 种最常用的模型是精益、改进模型、六西格玛和经验的共同设计。
- There are similar underlying principles in all models of improvement; the difference is the focus of emphasis within each model.
  所有改进模型都有相似的基本原则，只是每个模型聚焦的重点不同。
- Whether one single model is adopted, or a pick and mix approach is chosen, senior leaders need to be advocates of the chosen organisational approach to improvement for it to be successfully embedded.
  无论采用单一模式还是混合方法，高级领导都需要成为所选组织方法的倡导者，以便成功嵌入改进模型。

Introduction

As we have seen in Chapter 1, quality improvement thinking in healthcare has evolved from quality management practices in other industries, notably manufacturing. A range of quality improvement models have been developed from these practices and adapted over time. W. Edwards Deming (1900–1993) is often referred to as the 'Father of Quality Improvement' and his 14 principles of improvement ('14 Points for Management') have since been adopted as a foundation for all disciplines of improvement science. See Box 4.1.

It comes as no surprise, therefore, that there are similarities underpinning all the quality improvement philosophies and models that are prevalent in healthcare. These include the following:

- Liker's (2004) Toyota Way which is based on Ohno's (1988) Lean Production. This

引言

正如第 1 章所述，医疗保健质量改进思想从其他行业的质量管理实践发展而来，特别是制造业。从这些实践中开发了一系列质量改进模型，并随时间的推移进行了调整。爱德华兹·戴明（1900—1993 年）通常被称为"质量改进之父"，他的 14 条改进原则（也称为"14 个管理要点"）已经成为所有改进科学的学科基础。参见框 4.1。

因此，医疗保健领域的质量改进理念和模型相似之处就不足为奇了。包括以下内容：

- 莱克描述以大野（1988 年）精益生产为基础的丰田方式（2004 年）。这种方法的重点是从客户（或患者）的角度充分理解价值，然后创建持续改进的

Box 4.1 Principles of improvement.
框 4.1 **改进的原则**

1 Create constancy of purpose for improvement.
创造持续不变的改进目标。

2 Adopt the new philosophy.
采用新的理念。

3 Cease dependence on inspection to achieve quality.
不再靠检查来达到质量标准。

4 Work with a single supplier to reduce cost.
与单一供应商合作以降低成本。

5 Improve every process and service, constantly.
不断改进每个流程和服务。

6 Institute on the job training.
职业培训。

7 Improve leadership.
改进领导力。

8 Drive out fear.
驱除恐惧。

9 Break down silos.
打破孤岛。

10 Eliminate slogans, exhortations and targets for the workforce.
为员工消除口号、劝诫和目标。

11 Eliminate numerical quotas for the workforce and numerical goals for management.
取消绩效指标。

12 Remove barriers that rob people of pride in their workmanship.
消除对工作技能的不自信。

13 Institute a vigorous programme of education and selfimprovement for everyone.
为每个人制订合适的教育和自我改进方案。

14 Involve all workers in the transformation.
让所有员工参与转型。

Source: Deming (1982).
来源：戴明（1982 年）。

---

approach focuses on fully understanding value from the customer (or patient) perspective and then creating a continuous improvement approach to improve process and reduce 'waste'.

- Langley's (1996) Model for Improvement which focuses on small incremental improvement steps to reduce errors.
- Carey's (2001) continuous measurement of quality improvement based on Six Sigma methdology and Statistical Process Control (SPC), which focuses on understanding variation in outcome and in reducing

方法来改进流程并减少"浪费"。

- 兰利的改进模型（1996 年），侧重于小的渐进式改进步骤以减少错误。
- 凯里的基于六西格玛方法学和统计过程控制（SPC）质量改进的连续测量（2001 年），其重点在于理解结果的变异和减少变异。

variation.

The differences between approaches are subtle and relate to focus or emphasis; that is, which of the common core improvement principles are brought to the fore. These include a customer focus (Lean), collaborative problemsolving (Model for Improvement) or understanding variation (Six Sigma).

Healthcare organisations in the UK are learning from successful organisations in other parts of the world and are increasingly adopting an organisational approach to continuous quality improvement. Organisation-wide deployment of continuous improvement principles engages frontline staff and embeds a scalable methodology for growing and coordinating improvement activities. This approach is fast becoming an expectation of commissioners and regulators of healthcare and, as a result, many organisations have built improvement and transformation teams with specific expertise in their chosen methodology. Organisations such as the Virginia Mason Institute in the USA, Jonkoping County Council in Sweden, Southcentral Foundation in Alaska and Salford Royal NHS Foundation Trust in the UK have demonstrated that an organisation-wide approach to quality improvement, adopting a single model approach, creates a sustainable culture of improvement which benefits patient experience and the delivery of safe care.

This chapter now describes the four most common approaches to quality improvement used in healthcare organisations.

Lean

The most common model to be adopted as an organisation-wide approach in healthcare is 'Lean', based on the Toyota Production System. The appeal of this methodology to the healthcare context was the prevailing philosophy within Toyota about empowering frontline workers to improve processes in order to develop an enhanced and more effective product. In essence, Lean is the continuous and systematic elimination of waste, with waste being defined as anything that does not add value to the patient or process. Lean methodology describes five key tasks that, if addressed, deliver what the customer wants, and needs, at the highest quality and safety level possible with the lowest

各方法之间的差异是微妙的，与焦点或重点有关，也就是说，其核心改进相同，这些包括以客户为中心（精益）、协作解决问题（改进模型）及理解变化（六西格玛）。

英国的医疗机构正向世界其他地区的成功组织学习，并越来越多地采用组织方法来持续提高质量。在整个组织范围内部署持续改进原则使一线员工参与进来，并嵌入可扩展的方法来发展和协调改进活动。这种方法正迅速成为医疗专员和监管机构的心头好，因此，许多组织已经建立了改进和转型团队，他们在选择方法上具有特定的专业知识。美国弗吉尼亚梅森研究所、瑞典延雪平县议会、阿拉斯加中南部基金会和英国索尔福德皇家国家医疗服务体系基金会等组织已经证明，在整个组织范围内采用单一模型方法进行质量改进的方法，可创建一种可持续的改进文化，从而有益于患者体验和安全护理。

本章介绍医疗机构使用的 4 种最常见的质量改进方法。

精益

在医疗领域，组织范围内采用的最普遍的模式是基于丰田公司生产系统的精益方法。这种方法是丰田内部普遍的理念，即授权一线工作人员改进流程，以开发增强型和更有效的产品，对医疗行业有很大的吸引力。实质上，精益会不断消除系统性浪费，"浪费"被定义为对患者或流程没有增加价值的一切东西。精益方法描述了 5 项关键任务，如果得到解决，就能够让高度积极的员工用最低的成本和尽可能高的质量及安全水平为客户提供想要的东西（图 4.1）。

associated costs, provided by a highly motivated workforce. See Figure 4.1.

Applying the principles of Lean to healthcare brings to light what adds value from the patient's perspective and what does not. Value in Lean is defined by the patient. Any task or activity that is not a value-added step from the perspective of the patient is deemed wasteful, and eliminated. This immediately improves flow in the healthcare setting, relieves staff of the burden of unnecessary work, helps to improve the patient experience and, consequently, has a positive impact for the whole organisation (Figure 4.2). An example of the application of Lean methodology is provided in Box 4.2.

There are many documented examples that demonstrate where Lean has improved patient satisfaction, reduced waiting times and improved productivity. Improvements have also been recorded in processing paperwork and scheduling appointments. Health services have successfully deployed Lean in various areas of their operational processes but increasingly the approach is being adopted across whole organisations. One notable example where Lean has been adopted wholesale is by the US hospital and integrated care system, Virginia Mason. The Virginia Mason Institute is now supporting several Trusts in the UK to adopt a Lean approach.

将精益原则应用于医疗保健，从患者的角度揭示什么有用，什么无用，精益价值由患者定义。从患者的角度来看，一切不能让任务或活动增值的步骤都是浪费，应该消除。这立即改善了医疗机构的流动性，减轻了员工不必要的工作负担，有助于改善患者体验，从而对整个组织产生积极影响（图 4.2）。框 4.2 提供了应用精益方法的一个例子。

有许多记录下来的例子表明精益方法可以提高患者满意度，减少等待时间并提高生产力。在处理病历和安排预约方面也有改进的先例。卫生服务机构已经成功地将精益部署在其运营流程的各个方面，越来越多的方法正被整个组织采用。美国弗吉尼亚梅森医院综合护理系统就是大规模采用精益方法的一个例子，弗吉尼亚梅森医院现在正帮助英国的多个信托基金布署精益方法。

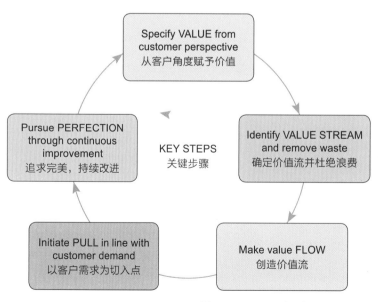

Figure 4.1 Lean: five key steps.

图 **4.1**　精益：5 个关键步骤

	STANDARD WORK 标准作业	REMOVE WASTE 杜绝浪费	VISUAL MANAGEMENT 可视化管理	ELIMINATE BATCHING 杜绝集中处理	IDENTIFY ROOT CAUSE 确定根本原因
What? 是什么?	Standard work enables the same processes to be followed whoever is undertaking the process 以标准作业执行该流程的任何人都可以遵循相同的流程	Identify what parts of the process are not adding value 确定哪些流程步骤无用	Develop a visual cue so that it is easy to see at a glance 设置一目了然的可视化提示	Undertake the process when the customer needs it rather than batching a lot together 在客户需要时处理, 而不是集中处理	Understand what is the main cause of the problem and fix that–rather than the symptom 通过了解问题的主要原因来解决问题, 而不是细节
How? 如何做?	Develop checklists and standard operating procedures that everyone follows 制订检查表, 确保每个人都遵循标准操作程序	Complete a process mapping exercise to identify where there is duplication and non-value added process steps 完成流程映射练习, 以确定重复和无用的流程步骤		Process requests as they come in rather than every week or month as this will reduce queues. Understand where the bottlenecks are and focus improvement in these areas 及时处理需求, 而不是集中处理每周或每月的需求, 因为这将减少堆积。了解瓶颈所在, 并将改进重点放在这些方面	Use the 5 why' to understand what the root cause is 用 5 个 "为什么" 来理解根本原因
Examples 示例	WHO Theatre Checklis 世卫组织手术室检查表 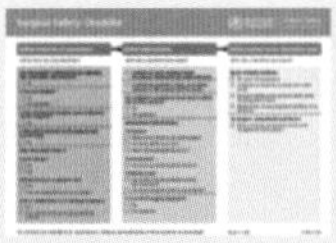	Value Stream map 价值流图 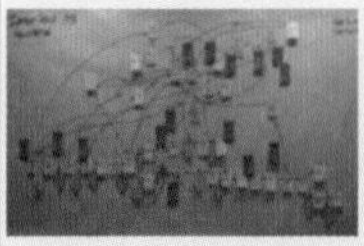	Kanban Cues 提示板 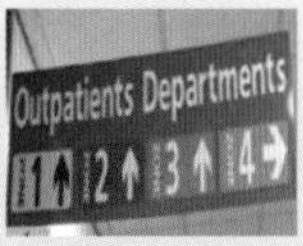	Daily rather than weekly referral management 每天而不是每周进行转诊管理 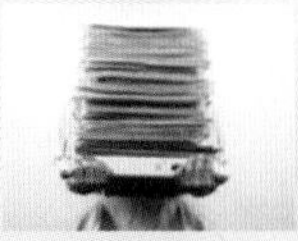	5 Why's? 5 个 "为什么" 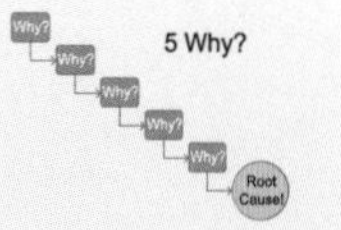
			Outpatients Departments 1 2 3 4		5 Why? Root Cause!

Figure 4.2 Lean interventions.
图 4.2 精益干预

Model for Improvement

The Model for Improvement (Langley et al., 2009) was originally developed by the Institute of Healthcare Improvement (IHI) in the USA and provides a relatively simple framework for delivering change at pace (Figure 4.3). The model is based on asking three fundamental questions to clarify the problem, understand what will be different if the change has been a success and to clarify the actual change required. It then goes on to provide a framework, known as a Plan Do Study Act (PDSA) cycle, for testing

改进模型

改进模型（Langley 等, 2009 年）最初是由美国医疗保健改进研究所（IHI）开发的, 它提供了一个相对简单的框架, 用于快速实现变革（图 4.3）。该模型基于提出的 3 个基本问题来阐明问题, 即如果变革成功会有什么不同, 并阐明想要的变革目标。然后, 它继续提供一个框架, 称为计划 - 执行 - 研究 - 行动（PDSA）循环, 用于测试变革和

Box 4.2 **Example: Reducing waiting times using Lean methodology.**
框 4.2   **示例：使用精益方法减少等待时间**

A psychology department was struggling to manage the number of referrals that were being received and new patients were not receiving appointments for many months. The reception staff were often phoned by patients who had been referred, but had not received an appointment and the psychology team were feeling very pressured – they knew patients weren't getting the best service and the management team kept telling them that they were failing waiting time expectations.

心理科全力管理转诊患者，新患者几个月内都无法预约。已经转诊但没有预约的患者经常会给接待人员打电话，心理团队的压力非常大，他们知道患者没有得到最好的服务，但管理团队不断告知，计划时间没有预约。

Lean methodology was introduced into the department. The team worked together to draw the process map and through doing this identified areas where there was waste, there was duplication, lots of patients were failing to attend appointments wasting new patient slots and reception staff were spending more time answering patient complaint calls about appointment times than arranging appointments.

该部门引入精益方法。团队合作绘制流程图，通过绘制流程图，确定了浪费、重复的步骤，许多患者未能预约，浪费了新患者的时间，接待人员在回答患者关于预约时间的投诉电话上花费的时间比安排预约的时间要多。

A new set of processes were developed with the team and working groups were set up to improve different aspects of the service. By the end of the project the waiting times for new patients had improved from 18 months to 12 weeks; staff were much happier, reception staff were using their time more effectively on booking appointments and supporting team activities and patient satisfaction with the booking process had improved significantly.

团队制订了一套新的程序，并成立了工作组，以改进服务的各个方面。到项目结束时，新患者的等待时间从 18 个月减少到 12 周；员工更快乐，接待人员更有效地利用时间预约和支持团队活动，患者对预约过程的满意度显著提高。

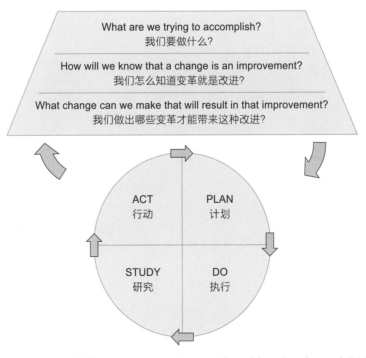

What are we trying to accomplish?
我们要做什么？

How will we know that a change is an improvement?
我们怎么知道变革就是改进？

What change can we make that will result in that improvement?
我们做出哪些变革才能带来这种改进？

ACT / 行动   PLAN / 计划
STUDY / 研究   DO / 执行

Figure 4.3 The Model for Improvement. Source: Adapted from Langley et al. (2009).
图 4.3   改进模型。资料来源：改编自兰利等（2009 年）

change(s) and reviewing impact (Box 4.3). You can find a detailed description of using PDSA cycles for developing and testing solutions in Chapter 8.

审查效果（框 4.3）。你可以在第 8 章中找到使用 PDSA 循环开发和测试解决方案的详细描述。

Box 4.3 **Example: Reducing long waits in hospital using the Model for Improvement.**
框 4.3　示例：使用改进模型减少住院时间

A hospital recognised that patients were staying in hospital for too long once they were medically fit for discharge. This was having an impact on patient well - being, with some patients getting sick again whilst waiting to leave hospital. Patients who needed a hospital bed were waiting too long in the emergency department because there was a shortage of acute medical beds available, and staff were becoming stressed at having to manage the continued pressure in the hospital.

一家医院发现，如果等到患者身体状况适合出院时再出院，那他们在医院的住院时间就太长了。这对患者的健康产生了影响，一些患者在等待出院过程中再次生病。需要病床的患者在急诊室等待的时间太长，因为急症病床不够用，工作人员不得不承受医院持续的压力。

The three questions of the Model for Improvement were considered:
考虑改进模型的 3 个问题：

What were we trying to accomplish?
我们想要达成什么？

A reduction in length of stay for our patients.
减少患者的住院时间。

How will we know if a change is an improvement?
我们如何知道变革是否是一次改进？

A reduction in the number of patients that stay in hospital over 21 days.
减少住院超过 21 天的患者数量。

What change can we make?
我们能够做出什么变革？

Ensure all patients have an active discharge plan that all the team follow.
确保所有患者的治疗团队都积极让患者出院。

PLAN Each ward in the project group was audited against a selection of best practice actions that have been proven to support a reduction in length of stay. The average length of stay on the ward and number of patients staying in hospital for more than 7 days, and more than 21 days was measured. Each ward then developed a plan for the next 7–14 days to achieve some level of change.

计划　项目组中的每个病房均制订了一系列最佳实践操作经审核，这些实践已被证明可缩短住院时间。采集了病房的平均住院时间和住院时间超过 7 天和超过 21 天的患者人数。然后，每个病房都制订了接下来 7~14 天的计划，以实现一定程度的变革。

DO Each of the wards implemented the plan over the following week.
执行　每个病房都在随后的 1 周实施了该计划。

STUDY The length of stay and numbers of patients staying over 7 and 21 days was monitored weekly. Staff satisfaction with the plan and patient experience was also measured. As was a balancing measure of the number of any readmissions.

研究　每周监测住院时间和住院超过 7 天和 21 天的患者人数，还测量了员工对该计划的满意度和其处理患者的经验度。这也是衡量重新入院人数的一项平衡措施。

ACT Wards shared with each other any progress or where things didn't work. Learning was shared and plans altered where things weren't making a difference. The PDSA cycle was then repeated over several months.

行动　病房之间互相分享进展或出现问题的地方。学习是共享的，在工作没有产生效果的地方对计划做出了改变。然后在几个月内重复 PDSA 循环。

RESULTS The number of patients staying over 21 days reduced as further PDSA cycles were implemented.
结果　随着 PDSA 循环的进一步实施，住院 21 天以上的患者人数减少了。

Six Sigma

Six Sigma is an improvement methodology focused on understanding variation and then reducing in-process variation to improve results. It is used to complement Lean methodology or can be used independently. Six Sigma has not been widely adopted in healthcare settings independently – perhaps because of cost, time constraints and its focus on the development of a small number of experts rather than mass participation by staff and/or patients – but where it is beneficial is in the focus on measurement and understanding variation.

The difference between Lean and Six Sigma is a subtle but important one. Lean focuses on improving flow and reducing waste, Six Sigma focuses on reducing errors and reducing variation in processes. See Figure 4.4.

The Six Sigma methodology uses a five-stage process known as DMAIC.

- Define the problem.
- Measure the size of the problem.
- Analyse to determine the root cause.
- Improve by implementing solutions that will eliminate the root cause.
- Control by monitoring variation using tools such as Statistical Process Control.

六西格玛

六西格玛是一种改进方法，其重点是理解变异，然后减少过程中的变异以改进结果。它用来补充精益方法，也可以独立使用。六西格玛还没有被大规模独立地应用于医疗环境中——也许是因为成本、时间限制以及只有少数专家的关注、发展，而不是员工和/或患者的大规模参与——但它的好处在于关注测量和理解变异。

精益和六西格玛之间的区别微妙但重要。精益专注于改善流程和减少浪费，六西格玛专注于减少错误和流程中的变异（图 4.4）。

六西格玛方法采用了一种称为 DMAIC 的 5 阶段流程。

- 确定问题。
- 测评问题的大小。
- 分析确定根本原因。
- 通过实施消除根本原因的解决方案进行改进。
- 通过使用统计过程控制等工具控制监测变异过程。

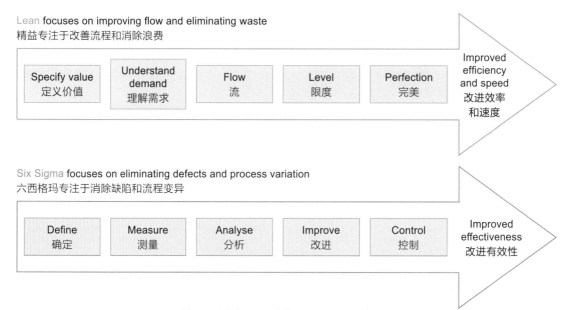

Figure 4.4 Lean and Sigma – a comparison.

图 4.4　精益与六西格玛的比较

Where Six Sigma is of benefit to healthcare is in the focus of understanding variation. Hospitals in the UK are increasingly using Statistical Process Control (SPC) Charts for performance monitoring as this tool provides more opportunity to understand the level of variation in a system. They enable the team to monitor improvement efforts and assist them in determining whether there is a marked sustainable change in performance or whether the change could be associated to natural variation within the system (Box 4.4).

医疗保健领域应用六西格玛的好处在于理解变异。英国的医院越来越多地使用统计过程控制图（SPC）进行业绩监控，因为这一工具提供了更多的机会来了解系统中的变异水平。它们使团队能够监控改进工作，并帮助确定业绩是否存在显著的可持续改变，或者这种改变是否与系统内的自然变异有关（框4.4）。

Box 4.4 Example: Improving discharge patterns using Six Sigma.

框 4.4 示例：使用六西格玛改进出院模式

A Trust recognised that the number of discharges at a weekend were significantly lower than the number of discharges during the week and so commenced a quality improvement project to reduce the level of variation that occurred between weekends and weekdays.

一家信托机构认识到，周末的出院人数明显低于1周内的出院人数，因此启动了1项质量改进项目，以减少周末和工作日之间出院人数的变化水平。

A Six Sigma methodology was deployed as follows:

六西格玛方法部署如下：

DEFINE The number of discharges on Saturday and Sunday are lower than Monday–Friday.

确定 星期六和星期天的出院人数低于星期一至星期五。

MEASURE Run charts were created to measure the number of discharges. See Figure 4.5.

测量 创建运行图来测量出院数，参见图4.5。

ANALYSE Patients that could potentially be medically fit and ready for discharge were not being reviewed routinely by doctors over the weekend as reduced capacity meant that doctors needed to focus on the sickest patients and those admitted over the weekend.

分析 医生没有在周末定期检查潜在的医学上健康并准备出院的患者，因为容量（床位）的减少意味着医生需要把重点放在最严重的患者和周末入院的患者身上。

IMPROVE A criteria-led discharge policy was written and implemented on four wards within the medical division with support of the clinical teams. Lead clinicians identified patients that would be suitable for discharge if certain clinical criteria were met at the weekends. This was documented in the patients notes and the nursing team were then able to discharge patients at the weekend, if the patient's clinical condition met the criteria identified in the plan. The discharge letter was pre-populated prior to the weekend to enable the medication to be requested from pharmacy and for the appropriate discharge correspondence to be completed.

改进 在临床团队的支持下，医疗部门的4个病房制定并实施了出院标准。主治医师确定如果周末存在符合某些出院标准的患者。如果患者的临床状况符合标准，护理团队就可以让其周末出院。出院信函是在周末之前预先填写的，以便能够从药房申请药物并完成出院告知。

CONTROL Weekend discharge rates continued to be monitored, as did readmission rates, in order to understand if patients returned to hospital more regularly following discharge via the new process. No evidence was found that readmission rates increased as a result; and discharge rates at a weekend began to increase.

控制 继续监测周末出院率和再入院率，以了解患者是否在通过新流程出院后能定期返回医院。没有证据表明再入院率因此而增加，同时周末的出院率开始上升。

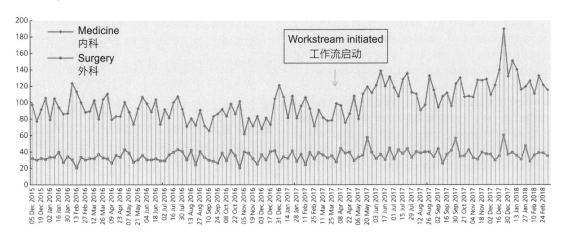

Figure 4.5 Example run chart – improving weekend discharge.

图 4.5　改进周末出院示例运行图

Traditionally in healthcare, performance has been measured using red/amber/green (RAG) charts to show where average performance over a period of time is hitting or not hitting a target. SPC charts support a deeper understanding of whether a reduction in performance on a particular day is the result of natural variation or if improvement focus could make a different to the performance. SPC run charts are described more fully in Chapter 9.

Experienced-based Co-design

Experience-based Co-design (EBCD) is a tool that was designed to develop simple solutions to improve patient experience. It uses a qualitative, story-telling approach that enables staff and patients to co-design services and care pathways together in partnership. It focuses on developing a deep understanding of how patients and staff experience a service. It does this by gathering the perspectives of patients and staff through in-depth interviewing, observations and group discussions. Emotionally significant points of the experience, known as key touch points, are then identified and the group assigns positive or negative feelings to each of these touch points.

A short, edited film is created from patient interviews. This is shown to staff and patients, conveying in an impactful way how patients experience the service. Staff and patients are then brought together to explore the findings and to work in small groups to identify and implement activities that will improve the service or the

传统上，在医疗保健领域，绩效是通过红 / 琥珀色 / 绿色（RAG）图表来衡量的，以显示一段时间内的平均绩效达到或未达到目标。SPC 运行图有助于更深入地了解某一天的业绩下降是自然变异的结果，还是集中在改进对绩效产生的影响。SPC 运行图在第 9 章中有更详细的描述。

基于体验的协同设计

基于体验的协同设计（EBCD）是一种旨在开发简单解决方案以改善患者体验的工具。它采用定性、讲故事的方法，使医护人员和患者能够合作设计服务和护理路径。它的重点是培养患者和医护人员对体验服务的深刻理解。通过深入访谈、观察和小组讨论，收集患者和员工的观点。然后确定体验中具有重要情感意义的点，即关键触点，然后小组为每一个触点分配正面或负面的情感。

给医护人员和患者播放了 1 个根据患者访谈制作的小短片，以有效的方式传达了患者对服务的体验。然后，医护人员和患者会聚在一起探讨研究结果，并分组进行工作，以识别和实施可改进的服务或护理途径。

care pathway.

Within healthcare, the approach has already been used in a range of clinical services, including cancer, diabetes, drug and alcohol treatment, emergency services, genetics, inpatient services, intensive care, mental health, orthopaedics, palliative care and surgical units (Box 4.5). Further information on the method can be obtained through the Point of Care Foundation (www.pointofcarefoundation.org. uk).

Single method vs 'pick and mix'

There is growing evidence that organisations that have committed to, and invested in, a single improvement approach have built significant momentum in their improvement journey. These organisations have developed training

在医疗保健领域，这一方法已被用于一系列临床服务，包括癌症、糖尿病、药物和酒精成瘾治疗、急救服务、遗传学、住院服务、重症监护、心理健康、骨科、姑息治疗和外科病房（框 4.5）。有关该方法的更多信息可通过尖端护理基金会获得 (www.pointofcarefoundation.org.uk)。

单一方法与"挑选和混合"

越来越多的证据表明，致力于应用单一改进方法的组织在其改进过程中逐渐积累了显著的动力。这些组织制订了培训计划，并

Box 4.5 Example: Improving outpatients using Experience-based Co-design.

框 4.5 示例：使用基于体验的协同设计改进门诊

An orthopaedic team were aware that there was opportunity to improve productivity, reduce the number of patients that did not attend for their appointment and reduce the number of complaints that were being received. They chose to use an Experience based Co-design methodology to understand what improvements could be made.

骨科团队想要提高生产力，减少没有预约的患者人数和收到的投诉数量。他们使用基于体验的协同设计方法来探索可以进行哪些改进。

An initial observation was undertaken to understand the key touch points in the patient journey (e.g. receiving referrals, sending appointment letters, receiving telephone calls regarding appointments, attending appointments, etc.) and to determine what areas would be beneficial to explore within the video interviews with both patients and staff.

初步观察，了解患者就医过程中的关键触点（如接受转诊、发送预约信、接收有关预约的电话、参加预约等），并确定哪些方面对患者和工作人员的视频访谈有利。

Patients and staff were invited to be involved in the co-design improvement exercise. This involved interviews, separate patient and staff feedback events, and then a joint feedback and improvement event to begin to design the improvement actions.

患者和工作人员共同参与设计改进活动。这包括面谈，单独的患者和医护人员反馈以及联合反馈和探讨改进方案，然后开始设计改进行动。

Initial interviews provided a wealth of data around the whole patient journey. Once data had been collated into key themes, separate feedback events allowed both staff and patients to explore the current challenges with the service and develop a map of experience.

最初的访谈提供了大量患者完整就医过程的数据。一旦将数据按重要主题加以整理，单独的反馈活动就可以让工作人员和患者探索当前的服务存在的问题，并开发出体验图。

Following the feedback events, staff and patients came together to develop improvement actions. Examples of improvement actions included a new appointment texting service, reviewing outpatient clinic templates to reduce the number of cancelled appointments, changing the layout of the waiting area, and information availability sent out with the appointments.

反馈之后，医护人员和患者一起制订改进措施，包括新的预约短信服务、设计预约门诊范例以减少取消预约的次数、更改等候区的布局以及发送预约信息。

programmes that staff are strongly encouraged to attend and, as a result, an improvement language becomes familiar across the organisation. In essence, these organisations are developing a culture of improvement – 'the way we do things round here' – which automatically generates further interest and engagement in the improvement methodology.

However, it is absolutely possible to intertwine the models described above. For example, by using Experienced-based Co-design to fully understand the patient experience and understand where the focus of improvement needs to be, measuring outcomes through statistical process control charts to understand the variation and monitor any impact of change, using process mapping tools from Lean methodology to identify where the waste in the process is, and developing PDSA cycles to test the changes identified. See Box 4.6.

For organisations to fully benefit from quality improvement activities there needs to be clear support and demonstrable involvement from leaders in the organisation. Senior leaders need to be advocates of the chosen method of improvement and can demonstrate this by being active sponsors of quality improvement programmes, engaging in the development of the improvement strategy, attending training programmes in the methodology and applying the methodology to their own processes. Alongside, a governance structure needs to be established that supports and maintains a culture of continuous improvement.

积极鼓励员工参加，因此，整个组织都熟悉改进语言。本质上，这些组织正在发展一种改进的文化——"我们在这里做事的方式"，这自然会让医护人员对改进方法产生更多的兴趣和参与。

然而，将上述模型交织在一起是绝对可能的。例如，通过使用基于经验的共同设计来充分了解患者体验和改进的重点，通过统计过程控制图来测量结果，理解变异并监控变革的所有影响，使用精益方法中的流程映射工具来确定流程中的浪费在哪里，并开发PDSA循环来测试既定的变革（框4.6）。

为了让组织从质量改进活动中充分受益，需要组织领导者的明确支持和大力参与。高级领导需要成为所选择的改进方法的倡导者，并且可以通过积极发起质量改进方案、参与改进战略的制定、参加方法学培训以及将方法应用于自己的流程来证明这一点。此外，还需要建立治理结构，以支持和保持持续改进的文化。

Box 4.6 **Choosing a model for improvement.**
框 4.6 **选择改进模型**

Model 模型	Requirements for success 成功的要求	When to use 何时使用
Lean 精益	Requires significant knowledge of the methodology and so, usually, Lean training is provided for employees before the organisation engages in using this approach Improvement activities are usually kickstarted within events such as week-long Rapid Improvement events with the expectation that continued improvement actions occur and are measured at 30, 60 and 90 day intervals 需要大量的方法学知识，因此，通常在组织使用这种方法之前会为员工提供精益方法培训 改进活动通常以周为周期快速，并且每隔 30 天、60 天和 90 天进行一次测量	Lean should be seen as a long-term solution to developing an organisational culture rather than a short-term change programme It can support the development of a culture where improvement is one of the fundamental tasks of every employee Lean is a useful approach to changing processes within and across pathways, known sometimes as going 'narrow and deep' 精益方法应该被视为发展组织文化的长期解决方案，而不是短期变革计划 它可以支持组织文化的发展，在这种文化中，改进是每个员工的基本任务 精益是一种有用的方法，可以改变途径内和跨界流程，有时称为"窄而深"
PDSA 计划-执行- 研究-行动	Requires and supports the engagement of people who are using the current process and enables them to be involved in testing the changes and informing on whether the test worked or requires further improvements before being implemented fully 要求和支持正在使用当前流程的人员参与，并让他们能测试变革，在完全实施之前告知测试是否有效或需要进一步改进	PDSA improvement cycles can be used to test improvements on a small scale before wider implementation of a new process PDSA 改进循环可用于更广泛地实施新流程之前测试小范围的改进
Six Sigma 六西格玛	Requires a deep understanding of the methodology and statistical expertise to analyse and interpret the data 需要深入了解分析和解释数据的方法与统计学知识	Six Sigma is helpful if there is significant variation within a process 六西格玛可以帮助发现流程中显著的变异
Experience based Co-design 基于体验的协同设计 （EBCD）	Requires a high level of interview and facilitation skills to develop a full picture of the current process from different perspectives. Patients and staff need a high level of support through the process, but it is an extremely valuable and worthwhile approach as the improvement actions are more likely to be successful due to the level of engagement required 高水平的访谈和协助技巧能从不同角度全面了解当前流程。患者和员工在整个过程中需要高度参与，这是一种非常有价值的方法，由于对参与者有要求，改进措施更有可能获得成功	The above methods should all have an element of staff and patient involvement for the processes to be redesigned effectively, however EBCD enables a much deeper level of patient and staff involvement and design in the improvement by focusing on patient and staff stories and understanding emotional touch points throughout the pathway 上述方法都需要员工和患者参与，以便重新有效地设计流程。然而，EBCD 通过关注患者和员工的故事并理解整个路径中的情感触点，使患者和员工参与和设计的层次更深

References
参考文献

Carey RG and Lloyd RC. (2001) *Measuring Quality Improvement in Health Care: A Guide To Statistical Process Control Applications*, Milwaukee, WI, American Society for Quality.

Deming WE. (1982) *Out of the Crisis*, Cambridge, MA, MIT Press.

Langley GL, Moen R, Nolan KM et al. (2009) *The Improvement Guide: A Practical Approach to Enhancing Organizational Performance*, San Francisco, Jossey - Bass.

Liker JK. (2004) *The Toyota Way: 14 Management Principles from the World's Greatest Manufacturer*, New York, McGraw - Hill.

Ohno T. (1988) *Toyota Production System: Beyond Large-Scale Production*, Cambridge, MA, Productivity Press.

Further reading and resources
深度阅读与相关资源

Bicheno J. (2008) *The Lean Toolbox for Service Systems*, Buckingham, PICSIE Books.

Graban M. (2016) *Lean Hospitals*, 3 edn, BocaRaton, FL, CRC Press.

Mann D. (2015) *Creating a Lean Culture. Tools to Sustain Lean Conversations*, BocaRaton FL, CRC Press.

NHS Improvement. *Making Data Count*. Available at: https:// improvement.nhs.uk/resources/making-data-count (accessed 23 September 2019).

NHS Improvement. *Improvement Hub*. Available at: https:// improvement.nhs.uk/improvement-hub/ (accessed 23 September 2019).

The Health Foundation (2013) *Improving Patient Flow*. Available at: https://www.health.org.uk/publications/ improving-patientflow (accessed 23 September 2019).

Womack J and Jones D. (2007) *Lean Solutions*, London, Simon & Schuster.

第 5 章 | 让人们加入

Lourda Geoghegan

Director of Improvement and Medical Director, Regulation and Quality Improvement Authority, Northern Ireland, UK

OVERVIEW
概述

- A shared understanding of the nature of the problem is a fundamental requirement to the success of any improvement activity.
  对问题性质的相同理解是改进活动成功的基本要求。

- Articulating the vision creates a picture of a future that people will want to buy in to.
  阐明愿景创造了一幅人们所希冀的未来蓝图。

- A collaborative approach means that many people working together on a problem are smarter and more capable than one person on their own.
  协作意味着许多人在一起解决 1 个问题比 1 个人更聪明、更有能力。

- A stakeholder analysis will inform a plan for engagement with others throughout the life of the work.
  利益相关者分析将明确整个工作周期内与他人合作的计划。

- Effective communication of any improvement activity is enhanced by combining data with narrative.
  通过将数据与叙述相结合,加强改进活动的有效沟通。

Identifying the problem together

Improving the quality of health and care delivered to patients and service users is a core element of professional practice for all staff, including those working in frontline services and across healthcare systems. Recognising a challenge as it exists, or as it becomes evident, in a care setting or through a patient's experience, is the first step on the quality improvement journey.

In practical terms, a quality challenge is frequently framed as a 'problem' and a solution or set of solutions is sought to address it. Complex health and care environments can give rise to many and varied problems, there is much literature on the types of problem occurring (critical, tame, wicked) and the types of response required for each problem (elegant and/or messy solutions) (Grint, 2008). Evidence indicates that

共同识别问题

改进向患者和服务用户提供的医疗和护理质量是所有医护人员(包括在一线服务和在医疗系统中工作的其他人员)专业实践的核心要素。在护理环境中或通过患者的经历认识到问题或问题已经很明显,是质量改进的第 1 步。

在实践中,"质量挑战"通常被定义为"问题",需要 1 个或 1 组解决方案来解决。复杂的医疗保健环境可能会导致许多不同的问题,关于问题的类型(严重、温和、奇怪)以及每个问题所需反应类型(优雅和 / 或混乱的解决方案)的文献很多(Grint,2008 年)。有证据表明,"一刀切"的方法是行不通的。

a 'one-size fits all' approach does not work.

Many factors will influence and contribute to the success of an improvement project or prototype, but the common requirement across all is gaining a shared understanding of the perceived problem, from the earliest opportunity. The individual improvement practitioner will actively seek out the views of people with a connection to the problem and the situation or context in which the problem is identified. They will take time to meet and engage with people who will be invited to talk about the problem from their own perspective (see Box 5.1).

This approach intentionally uses others' perspectives to build a shared understanding of the nature of the problem. It enables improvers to think differently, to hear and use different

许多因素会影响和促进改进项目或原型的成功，但所有这些因素都要求尽早就达成对问题的一致看法。从事改进工作的人要积极征求问题相关者的意见以及发现问题的情景或环境，花时间与从角度讨论问题的人见面对方的互动（框 5.1）。

这种方法有意利用他人的观点来建立对问题本质的共识。它使改进者能够以不同的方式思考，倾听和使用不同的语言，以不同的方式描述挑战，重新思考问题。通过这一过程，出现了新的想法，产生了解决问题的新的可能性。

Box 5.1 **Obtaining perspectives: people who can contribute.**
框 5.1　**获取观点：可以做出贡献的人**

- Team members from practitioner's own team.
  改进者自己团队的成员。
- Clinical colleagues.
  - practitioner's service.
  - wider multidisciplinary team.
  - special interest or experience.
  临床同事。

  ——改进者的服务机构。

  ——广泛的跨学科团队。

  ——特殊兴趣或经验。
- Patients and service users.
  患者和服务用户。
- Family members and carers.
  家人和照顾者。
- Advocacy and support groups.
  倡改和支持团体。
- Administration and management colleagues.
  负责行政和管理的同事。
- Wider health and care system.
  - improvement advisor and team.
  - commissioning and planning teams regulator.
  更广泛的医疗保健体系。

  ——改进顾问和团队。

  ——调试和规划团队。
- Outside health and care (e.g. similar improvement in different context).
  医疗护理之外（例如，在不同背景下的类似改进工作）。

language, to describe the challenge in a different way and to reframe the problem in question. Through this process new ideas emerge and new possibilities to address the problem are generated.

Early engagement provides the practitioner with an opportunity to begin work on the relational aspects of the improvement(s) they will either deliver themselves or facilitate others to deliver. Actions to engage early with others, to seek and hear others' perspectives and to reframe the problem help the practitioner to make sense of what is happening in their particular healthcare environment. These actions are important early signals from the practitioner to colleagues and interested parties that they will work collaboratively; the practitioner is shifting away from 'I know about this and I have all the solutions' to 'we have a shared understanding of the problem and together we will design the solutions'.

Key to this early engagement is that the improvement practitioner adopts an open and an inquisitive approach, they are curious throughout, they ask open questions and continue to refine their personal skills in 'formulating and asking the right question'. A questioning culture will encourage thinking and stimulate solutions to even the most complex of problems.

Articulating the vision and benefits

Having taken time to engage and obtain others' perspectives on the perceived problem, the task now evolves, and the practitioner begins to think about what a vision for the future might be. A vision is a picture of the future with some explanation as to why people will or would want to achieve that future. The vision for the improved state will describe a future in which the identified problem is addressed to a greater or lesser degree depending on the circumstance. The vision will make reference to parties or people for whom the improvement is relevant and important. Box 5.2 summarises why a clear vision is important.

In creating an effective vision, the improvement practitioner will work through a number of stages, continuing to adopt a highly collaborative approach. They may have penned an early blueprint of the vision, informed by their personal interest and early engagements, and

尽早参与可以为改进者提供一个机会，他们可以在自己实现或促进他人实现改进的相关方面着手进行工作。尽早与他人接触、寻求和倾听他人的观点并重新审视问题，有助于改进者理解在他们在特定的医疗环境中发生的事情。这些行动是改进者向同事和相关方发出的早期重要信号，表明他们将协同工作；改进者正在从"我知道这一点，我有所有的解决方案"转变为"我们对问题看法相同，我们将共同设计解决方案"。

早期参与的关键在于，改进实践者采用开放和探究的方法，他们始终保持好奇心，提出开放性问题，并不断完善"提出正确问题"的技能。质疑文化会鼓励思考，激发出解决最复杂问题的方法。

阐明愿景和收益

花时间讨论并获得他人对所感知问题的观点后，任务开始发生变化，改进者开始思考未来的愿景可能是什么。愿景是对未来的描绘，并对人们为什么想要实现这一未来做一些说明。在这个构思的未来中，所确定的问题将根据具体情况得到或多或少的解决。愿景将涉及与改进相关且重要的组织和人员。框 5.2 总结了愿景清晰的重要性。

在创建一个有效的愿景时，改进实践者将经历多个阶段，继续采用高度协作的方法。他们可能已经根据个人兴趣和早期参与情况，起草了愿景的早期蓝图，这应该作为迭代过程的一部分，并与利益相关者分享，以促进讨论和激发思考。每一次迭代都将提供一个

> **Box 5.2 Why a clear vision for improvement is important.**
>
> **框 5.2   为什么清晰的改进愿景很重要**
>
> A clear vision for improvement:
>
> 一个清晰的改进愿景：
>
> - Explicitly states what the improved future will look like.
>   明确指出改进后的未来会是什么样。
> - Underpins the strategy and plan to deliver the improvement.
>   为实现改进奠定战略和计划的基础。
> - Motivates people to take action(s) aligned to the improved future.
>   激励人们采取与改进后的未来相一致的行动。
> - Helps co-ordinate the actions of people who are working on the improvement.
>   帮助协调改进人员的行动。

this should be shared with stakeholders as part of an iterative process, to prompt discussion and stimulate thinking. Each iteration will provide an opportunity to shape the overall vision for the work. Evidence indicates that both 'the head and the heart' are required: the practitioner will need to employ both analytical and relational skills throughout this process.

The practitioner should expect to take time to facilitate work on creating an effective vision; this is rarely achieved through a single meeting. The benefit that patients, colleagues and other stakeholders will expect to receive from the work – that is, the advantage to be gained by each individual or group – should align with definition of the overall vision. The practitioner should systematically capture the expected high-level benefits for each individual or group, mapping these will further crystallise the vision under development.

You can read more on envisioning and participatory approaches to change in Chapter 12.

Involving the team and those who benefit

The landscape in which health and care is delivered is increasingly complex and challenging. There are many wicked problems, each requiring a different approach. Successful approaches rely not only on technical knowledge and individual capability but on skills in the relational and contextual domains of improvement. Collaboration is essential.

机会来塑造工作的整体愿景。证据表明，"大脑"和"心脏"都是必需的：改进者将需要在整个过程中同时运用分析技能和交往技巧。

改进者应该认识到创造有效愿景需要时间，很少能通过一次会议来实现。患者、同事和其他利益相关者期望从工作中获得的收益，即每个人或小组获得的收益应与总体愿景定义的一致。改进者应系统地捕捉每个人或小组的预期高水平收益，将其绘制出来，进一步使正在发展的愿景具体化。

你可以在第 12 章中阅读更多关于愿景和参与变革的方法。

让团队和受益者参与

提供保健和护理的环境越来越复杂，具有挑战性。有许多奇怪的问题，每一个都需要不同的方法。成功的方法不仅依赖技术知识和个人能力，而且还依赖关系和改进技能。合作是必不可少的。协作式领导基于这样一个原则：许多人在一起比 1 个人更聪明、更

Collaborative leadership is based on the principle that many people together are smarter and more capable than one on their own. The practitioner will work across boundaries to involve his/her team, patients and stakeholders. The conditions that optimise this engagement and influence success are summarised in Box 5.3.

There are many ways to involve people in the early stages of improvement. These range from short learning conversations, undertaken as and when an opportunity arises, to formal engagement events which are planned and facilitated. For the practitioner who identifies a problem in their local service or care setting and has an idea about how the problem can be improved, the practical approach is to start small and local – engage in early conversations, seek a variety of perspectives from all parts of the team or service and be open to learning through engaging with others.

Co-production is a partnership approach to developing and improving healthcare which brings people together to find shared solutions. In practice this involves partnering with people from the start to the end of any change or improvement that affects them. The practitioner will engage with a view to identifying people to co-design and co-deliver the improvement

有能力。改进者将跨界工作，让团队成员、患者和利益相关者参与进来。框 5.3 总结了成功组织队伍的要素。

有很多方法可以让人们在改进的早期阶段就参与进来，包括简短学习交流，到计划和促进参与正式活动。对于在当地服务或护理环境中发现问题并知道如何改进的改进者，实际的方法是从小规模和本地化开始，即尽早开展对话，从团队或服务机构的各个组织寻求各种观点，并通过与他人接触进行开放式学习。

协同生产是一种发展和改进医疗保健的合作方式，它将人们聚集在一起寻找解决方案。在实践中，这从始至终都需要与受到变革或改进影响的人进行合作。改进者将努力确定参与协同设计和共同交付所需改进的人员，从而超越传统的吸引、咨询或告知用户的方法。框 5.4 总结了支持协同生产方式的原则，框 5.5 总结了采用该方式的收益。

Box 5.3 Conditions to optimise engagement with team, patients and stakeholders.
框 5.3   团队、患者和利益相关者积极参与的要素

- A compelling shared vision for the future.
  对未来有共同的愿景。
- A shared commitment to work together over time.
  共同合作的长期承诺。
- Frequent contact between all involved to build trust and make real progress.
  所有相关人员频繁接触，以建立信任并取得实际进展。
- A shared contract to surface and resolve conflicts quickly, fairly, transparently and without blame.
  制订合同，以迅速、公平、透明及不受指责的方式使冲突浮出水面并予以解决。
- A commitment to collaborative problem solving.
  致力于通过协作解决问题。
- A commitment to shared learning for improvement rather than blame for mistakes.
  致力于分享学习成果以促进改进，而不是责怪他人的错误。
- A commitment to support and value each other and all participants.
  承诺给予彼此以及所有参与者支持与重视。
- Equal partnership between those working in health and care services and those who are served by these services.
  医务工作者与接受医疗服务的人之间建立平等的伙伴关系。

required, moving beyond the traditional approaches of engaging, consulting or informing service users. The principles underpinning a co-production approach are summarised in Box 5.4 and the benefits of adopting the approach are summarised in Box 5.5.

Box 5.4 Principles underpinning a co-production approach.

框 5.4　协同生产的基本原则

- Valuing people.

  对人的重视。
- Building representative networks.

  拓展人脉。
- Building people's capacity.

  培养人的能力。
- Reciprocal recognition.

  相互尊重。
- Cross-boundary working.

  跨界工作。
- Enabling and facilitating.

  给予便利。

Box 5.5 Benefits of adopting a co-production approach.

框 5.5　协同生产所获收益

- People's experience of care demonstrably improves.

  护理体验明显改进。
- People are empowered to take active responsibility for their health and well-being.

  公民有权对自己的健康和幸福承担积极责任。
- A strengths-based approach harnesses expertise and pools resources, talents and expertise.

  利用优势，汇集资源、人才和专业知识。
- Staff are proactively involved as partners, are empowered and take responsibility for improving outcomes.

  员工成为合作伙伴会积极参与，赋予其权力，他们也愿意对改进成果负责。

Communicating and engaging with stakeholders

与利益相关者沟通互动

Early in the improvement journey the practitioner will facilitate an analysis of the environment and context in which the work will be undertaken. This process is called a stakeholder analysis. It involves an assessment of the healthcare system and the changes under consideration as they relate to the main people or organisations in that system who have a vested interest. This analysis will inform a plan

　　在改进过程的早期，改进者将对工作环境和背景做分析。这个过程被称为利益相关者分析。它涉及对医疗体系的评估，以及尚在考虑中的变革，因为这些变革与医疗体系中的既得利益者或组织有关。该分析将在整个工作周期内为利益相关者接触提供信息。这种参与可能有几种形式：一些利益相关者

for engagement with stakeholders throughout the life of the work. This engagement may take several forms – some stakeholders may require a regular written report, while others may only require a verbal update at key stages – and it may help to define in advance the groups who may need more input than others. A stakeholder matrix, such as the one in Figure 5.1, may help to clarify who these are.

Engagement with stakeholders will require effective communication of the vision for the improvement work. The vision should be set out simply without jargon, include an example or analogy, be discussed at all relevant forums or meetings and be repeated as much as possible. The practitioner should be willing to engage in discussion of the content of the vision and to provide clarity if queries or inconsistencies arise.

Effective communication channels throughout the life of the improvement activity benefit from both formal feedback – for example, at planned meetings – and more informal opportunities for stakeholders to contribute their thoughts – for example, by email or telephone. Giving attention to how a more inclusive environment may be created means those involved can have the confidence of having their voice heard.

可能需要定期的书面报告，而另外一部分人可能只需要在关键阶段做口头，这有助于提前确定那些可能需要比其他人做出更多投入的群体。利益相关者矩阵如图 5.1 所示，有助于阐述这些人是谁。

与利益相关者接触时需要对改进工作的愿景做有效沟通。愿景应该简单，不使用行话，如举例子或类比，在所有相关论坛或会议上讨论，并尽可能重复。改进者应该参与对愿景的讨论，并在出现疑问或不一致时提供清晰的说明。

在改进活动的整个生命周期中，有效的沟通渠道既受益于正式反馈（例如在有计划的会议上），也受益于更多非正式的场合，让利益相关者贡献他们的想法（例如通过电子邮件或电话）。注重创造一个更具包容性的环境，意味着参与其中的人相信自己的声音能够被听到。

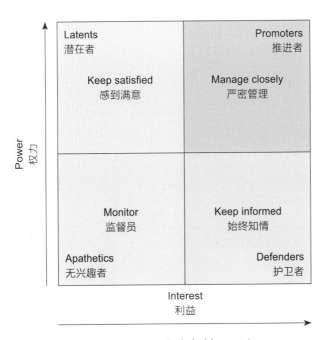

Figure 5.1 Stakeholder matrix.

图 5.1　利益相关者矩阵

Telling a compelling story

While facts and figures are important in communicating effectively, research indicates they are insufficient if used on their own and need to be accompanied by a compelling narrative; in effect, a story. Human beings are more likely to remember a fact if it's wrapped in a story. Stories have a stronger emotional impact than information presented quantitatively. For the practitioner seeking to bring people on board with their improvement, the story is essential; it requires thought and attention. The practitioner must use the story to engage, inspire and connect emotionally with the listener.

Engaging with patients and service users

All improvement efforts benefit from the unique insight and different perspectives that patients bring to the table, enhancing the chances that the improvement will build a service more aligned to patient and local needs. By involving them from the outset, patients can meaningfully partner in the design and implementation of the work and dissemination of any findings and the resultant changes made. It should be made clear how patients may get involved; for example, through consultation, partnership and/or patientled projects. Strategies to involve patients may include collecting patient experience data, recruiting patients opportunistically – for example, through existing personal contacts – recruiting patients with a particular condition or from membership of a pre-existing committee, inviting patients to participate in focus groups, recruiting a trained patient leader and/or developing a patient and service user advisory group (The Point of Care Foundation, 2013).

Summary

Getting people on board with any quality improvement activity is crucial to its success. Ensuring the early involvement of stakeholders in a variety of ways that harness meaningful collaboration will mean the full potential of the vision for improvement may be successfully and sustainably realised. Quality improvement practitioners must receive appropriate training. Time is well spent maximizing

讲一个引人注目的故事

虽然事实和数字在有效沟通中很重要，但研究表明，单独使用这些事实和数字是不够的，需要有令人信服的叙述，实际上需要一个故事。如果一个事实被包装在一个故事里，人类更容易记住它。故事比定量呈现的信息具有更强的情感关联。对于那些试图让人们参与改进的改进者来说，故事是必不可少的，它需要思考和关注。改进者必须用故事来吸引听众，启发他们，并在情感上与他们建立联系。

与患者和用户接触

所有的改进工作都得益于患者带来的独特见解和不同观点，这能够建立更符合患者和当地需求的服务。通过从一开始就让他们参与，患者可以富有意义地参与工作的设计和实施，散播事实和由此产生的变革。应明确患者如何参与，例如通过协商、建立伙伴关系和 / 或参与项目。让患者参与的策略包括收集患者体验数据、适时招募患者（例如通过现有的个人联系人）——招募具有特定病情的患者或从现有委员会的成员中招募患者、邀请患者参与重点小组，招募训练有素的患者领导和 / 或建立患者和用户咨询小组（尖端护理基金会，2013 年）。

总结

让人们参与质量改进活动对其成功至关重要。确保利益相关者以各种方式尽早参与，利用有意义的合作，将意味可以释放改进愿景的全部潜力并可持续地实现改进。质量改进工作者必须接受适当的培训。从患者体验中学习，倾听患者的声音，让患者参与协作

meaningful patient and carer involvement in quality improvement by learning from the patient experience, hearing the patient voice and engaging patients in collaboration and partnership and involving patients and carers in training improvement practitioners.

并建立伙伴关系，以及让患者和护理人员参与改进者的培训，能够充分利用时间，最大限度地提高患者和护理人员参与质量改进的意义。

References
参考文献

Grint K. (2008) Wicked problems and clumsy solutions: The role of leadership. *The New Public Leadership Challenge*, 1, 169-186.

The Point of Care Foundation (2013) *Experience-based Co-design Toolkit*. Available at: www.pointofcarefoundation.org.uk/ resource/experience-based-co-design-ebcd-toolkit/ (accessed 27 October 2019).

Further reading and resources
深度阅读与相关资源

Department of Health (NI) (2018) *Co-Production Guide for Northern Ireland-Connecting and Realising Value Through People*. Available at: www.health-ni.gov.uk/publications/coproduction-guide-northern-ireland-connecting-and-realisingvalue-through-people (accessed 9 September 2019).

Healthcare Improvement Scotland (2014) *Ready to Lead? Developing the Skills that Drive Change*. Available at: www. healthcareimprovementscotland.org/previous_resources/ implementation_support/ready_to_lead.aspx (accessed 9 September 2019).

Kotter J. (1996) *Leading Change*. Brighton, MA: Harvard Business School Publishing.

NHS Institute for Innovation and Improvement (2007) *Thinking Differently. Concepts, Tools and Methods to Unblock Thinking in Healthcare*. Available at: www.innovationagencynwc.nhs.uk/media/documents/PIP/thinking_differently%20Book%20(2). pdf (accessed 9 September 2019).

The Leadership Centre (2015) *The Art of Change Making*. Available at: www.leadershipcentre.org.uk/wp-content/uploads/2016/02/The-Art-of-Change-Making.pdf (accessed 9 September 2019).

第 6 章 | 识别问题

Ruth Glassborow

Director of Improvement, Healthcare Improvement Scotland, Edinburgh, UK

OVERVIEW
概述

- The way data is used to identify and diagnose improvement opportunities is different to the way data is used to understand if a change is leading to an improvement.
  数据用于识别和诊断改进时机与用于了解变革是否导致改进不同。
- A variety of data, both qualitative and quantitative, can be used to identify quality problems.
  各种定性和定量数据可用于识别质量问题。
- The use of benchmarking data is a common approach but one that, if misused, can drive poorer outcomes (Powell et al., 2003).
  使用基准数据是一种常见的方法，但如果使用不当，可能会导致较差的结果（Powell 等，2003 年）。
- It is important to include data from the patient's perspective.
  从患者的角度纳入数据很重要。
- Concepts from value-based healthcare can help in identifying problem areas as well as helping you think about which issue to address first.
  基于价值的医疗保健可以帮助确定问题所在的领域，并有助于考虑解决问题的优先级。

Using data to identify quality problems

Good use of data underpins all quality improvement work but the way that data is used to identify and diagnose improvement opportunities is different to the way data is used to understand if a change is leading to an improvement. This chapter focuses on using data to identify quality problems, the next chapter looks at using data to diagnose the improvement opportunity. Chapters 8 and 9 cover how to use data to understand if change is leading to an improvement.

There are broadly two types of data that are routinely used to identify quality problems:

- Quantitative (numerical) data, such as comparative (benchmarking) data and clinical audit data. This type of data is particularly useful for identifying an area of

利用数据识别质量问题

擅长使用数据是所有质量改进工作的基础，但使用数据来识别和诊断改进与了解变革是否导致改进不同。本章重点介绍如何使用数据识别质量问题，下一章将介绍如何使用数据确定改进时机。第 8 章和第 9 章介绍了如何使用数据来判断变革是否导致了改进。

通常有 2 种类型的数据可用于识别质量问题：

- 定量（数字）数据，如比较（基准）数据和临床审计数据。这类数据用于确定可以改进的实践领域特别好用。

practice where improvements could be made.

- Qualitative (descriptive) data, such as significant event analysis, complaints, patient and carer feedback and inspection reports. This type of data lends itself towards a more in-depth understanding of what problems may be driving poor-quality care.

Quantitative approaches

Using comparative data to identify opportunities for improvement

Comparing the performance of your team and/or service against other similar teams can highlight areas where your service could improve its performance. Any service committed to high-quality care should always be asking itself: 'who is the best in class at this and how do we compare'? Used badly, comparative benchmarking data can drive poorer outcomes and the following paragraphs highlight some of the common issues you need to address to ensure you make good use of comparative data.

Any ranked numerical list will have a top and a bottom. Key to effective use of comparative data is understanding whether the differences are statistically significant. A simple way of doing this which controls for differences in sample sizes is through the use of a funnel plot. Points above or below the funnel limits differ from the others by more than would be expected by chance. You can use it to identify units you might need to focus improvement work on – and also those which you might have something to learn from. An example is given in Figure 6.1.

Comparative data are widely used in health services to compare inputs. These are the resources which are needed to carry out a process or provide a service, such as staffing and number of inpatient beds. Looking at inputs in isolation of data on patient outcomes and overall costs can result in actions which make services worse. An example is given in Box 6.1.

Comparative data might tell you that improvement is possible, it doesn't on its own tell you how. So, key to effective use of comparative data is understanding what is driving the better performance in another system. Options for exploring this include looking at any published case studies and/or visiting the service yourself. Negotiating for a small group from your service to visit a better performing system

- 定性（描述性）数据，如重大事件分析、投诉、患者和护理者反馈以及检查报告。这类数据有助于更深入地了解哪些问题可能导致医疗质量低下。

定量方法

使用数据确定改进的时机

将团队和／或服务机构的绩效与其他类似团队进行比较，可以突出显示能够改进绩效的领域。任何致力于高质量护理的服务机构都应该扪心自问："谁在这方面是最好的，如何比较？"如果使用不当，比较基准数据可能会导致较差的结果，以下段落将重点介绍需要解决的常见问题，以确保充分利用比较数据。

所有排序的数字列表都有顶部和底部。有效利用比较数据的关键是了解差异是否具有统计学意义。控制样本大小差异的一种简单方法是使用漏斗图。高于或低于漏斗极限的点与其他点的差异超出了预期，可以使用它来确定可能需要集中改进的工作单元，以及可能需要从中学习的单元。图 6.1 给出了一个示例。

比较数据在医疗服务中被广泛用于比较投入。投入是指执行流程或提供服务所需的资源，如人员配置和住院病床数量。孤立地看待患者疗效和总体成本的数据，可能导致更糟的服务，参见框 6.1。

比较数据可能会告诉你改进是可能的，但它本身并不能告诉你如何改进。因此，有效利用比较数据的关键是了解是什么推动了另一个系统有更好的绩效。探索这一点可以查看所有已发表的案例研究和／或亲自访问服务机构。从服务机构中争取一小群人去访问一个表现更好的组织，有助于建立一种信念，即改进是可能的，从而有助于建立当地急需的变革意愿。如果你不能去拜访他们，

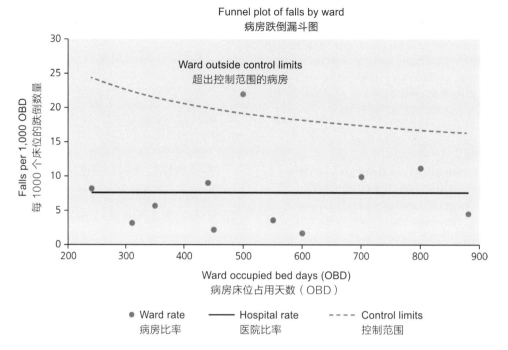

In this example, which looks at the rates of falls across eleven wards, only one of the eleven wards has a rate that makes it a statistically significant outlier. This means that, unlike the other wards, its higher falls rate is unlikely to be explained simply by normal random variation. An investigation into what the outlier ward is doing differently from the other wards is likely to highlight changes to behaviours and/or processes that, if implemented, would reduce the falls rate.

在这个例子中，观察了 11 个病房的跌倒率，11 个病房中只有 1 个病房的跌倒率是统计学上显著的异常值。这意味着，这个病房与其他病房不同，其较高的跌倒率不太可能简单地用正态随机变化来解释。调查离群病房与其他病房的不同之处，可能会突显出一些行为和 / 或流程的变革，如果实施这些变革，跌倒率将降低。

Figure 6.1 Example of a funnel plot.

图 6.1 漏斗图示例

Box 6.1 Using comparative data to compare inputs.

框 6.1 使用比较数据来比较成本

Benchmarking data highlights that Service A has statistically significant higher administrative costs than its comparators. However, a more detailed analysis finds that this has enabled the clinical staff to spend significantly less time on administration duties and hence treat a higher number of patients than other similarly staffed clinical teams. Further, an analysis of clinical outcomes shows it as a positive outlier. This wider analysis reveals that overall the service is both more effective and more cost efficient, in part because it has invested more in administrative resource.

基准数据表明，服务机构 A 的管理成本在统计学上显著高于其比较者。然而，更详细的分析发现，这让临床工作人员在行政事务上花费的时间显著减少，因此治疗的患者数量比其他类似人员配置的临床团队要多。此外，对临床结果的分析显示它是一个正的异常值。这一更广泛的分析表明，总的来说这个服务机构更有效，成本更低，部分原因是它在管理方面投入了更多资源。

can also have the benefit of creating a belief that improvement is possible, hence helping to create that much needed will for change locally. If you can't go and see them, consider arranging for them to come to visit and critique your system or arranging a webinar with them.

National clinical audits

One weakness of comparative data is that it only tells you how good you are compared with others and this can hide quality problems if performance is poor across all services. Clinical audit is a way to find out if healthcare is being provided in line with agreed quality standards.

National clinical audits assess performance against agreed quality standards while also providing, as a minimum, a current national average against which to benchmark local performance. National clinical audits are only available for a select number of conditions. In the UK, the National Clinical Audit and Patient Outcomes Programme (NCAPOP) are managed on behalf of NHS England by the Healthcare Quality Improvement Partnership (HQIP). The programme comprises more than 30 national audits related to some of the most commonly occurring conditions. Most of the projects involve services in England and Wales; some also include services from Scotland and Northern Ireland. You can find out more about the country specific programmes in Northern Ireland, Scotland and Wales by following the links provided at the end of this chapter.

Qualitative approaches

Significant event analysis (SEA)

In contrast to national clinical audits, which seek to enable learning from large sets of data, significant event analysis (significant events are also referred to as clinical incidents) is focused on investigating, reviewing and learning from a single event.

A significant event analysis (SEA) is defined by Pringle, Bradley and Carmichael (1995) as:

'A process in which individual episodes (when there has been a significant occurrence either beneficial or deleterious) are analysed in a systematic and detailed way to ascertain what can be learnt about the overall quality of care, and to indicate any changes that might lead to future improvements.'

可以考虑安排他们来参观和指导你的组织，或者安排网络研讨会。

国家临床审计

比较数据的一个缺点是，它只告诉您与其他人相比有多好，如果所有服务都很差，这可能会隐藏质量问题。临床审计是一种查明医疗保健是否符合质量标准的方法。

国家临床审计根据制订的质量标准评估绩效，同时提供至少一个当前的国家平均水平，以作为当地绩效的基准。国家临床审计仅适用于部分情况。在英国，国家临床审计和患者结果计划（NCAPOP）由医疗质量改善伙伴关系（HQIP）代表英国国家医疗服务体系（NHS）管理。该方案包括 30 多项国家审计，涉及最常见的一些情况。大多数服务项目涉及英格兰和威尔士；还包括来自苏格兰和北爱尔兰的一些服务。通过本章末尾提供的链接，您可以了解更多有关北爱尔兰、苏格兰和威尔士国家特定计划的信息。

定性方法

重大事件分析（SEA）

与寻求从大数据中获取信息的国家临床审计不同，重大事件（又称临床事件）分析侧重于调查、审查和从单个事件中了解。

普林格尔、布拉德利和卡迈克尔（1995年）将重大事件分析（SEA）定义为：

"以系统和详细的方式分析个别事件（当发生有益或有害的重大事件时）的流程，以确定对整体护理质量的了解，并指出可能导致未来改进的任何变革。"

This definition is inclusive of learning from what goes unusually well but, in practice, SEA is mainly applied to learning from a situation where something has gone wrong. Done well, a SEA involves all relevant members of the multidisciplinary care team and provides a structured process and a safe space to consider the range of factors that may have contributed to the event and identifying where improvement efforts may then be focused. This means it can also contribute towards creating learning cultures which are conducive to delivering and continuously improving care. However, a risk of SEAs is that, unless the recommendations are fed into a clear process for prioritising quality improvement activity, they can result in resources being directed at mitigating the risk of a rare event without sufficient consideration of whether those same resources could have a higher impact if focused on more common quality problems.

Complaints and feedback data

Complaints and feedback can be a rich source of information about quality issues in your system. Good investigation processes will drill into the root causes of complaints, recognising that the issue complained about is often a symptom of a poorly functioning system. Contributory factors often include unclear processes and roles, lack of availability of appropriately skilled professionals and/or equipment and/or a culture which stifles quality and learning. Without this root cause analysis there is a risk that you focus your improvement work on the wrong issues; for instance, re-training staff when the problem is not with their skills but with the time available to do everything that is being required. Ideally you want to go beyond complaints and actively seek feedback about what is and isn't working from both patients and staff.

User research

User research takes you beyond simple feedback and helps you to understand the experiences, needs, behaviours and motivations of those using your service. It can provide valuable insights for designing services which better meet user needs. In the healthcare context, users include patients and carers. However, when thinking about opportunities to improve your

这个定义包括从异常顺利的事情中学习，但在实践中，SEA 主要用于从发生错误的情况中学习。做得好的 SEA 涉及多学科护理团队的所有相关成员，并提供了一个结构化的流程和安全的空间来考虑可能导致事件的因素，并确定改进工作的重点。这意味着它也有助于创造利于改进的护理学习文化。然而，SEA 的一个风险是，除非将建议纳入明确的质量改进活动优先顺序的流程中，否则它们可能导致资源耗费于降低罕见事件的风险，而没有充分考虑这些资源如果集中在更常见的质量问题上是否会产生更大的影响。

投诉和反馈数据

投诉和反馈是系统中有关质量问题广泛的信息来源。良好的调查流程将从根本上带动深入调查投诉，认识到投诉的问题往往意味着系统运行不良。通常包括流程和角色不明确、缺乏适当技能的专业人员、设备或扼杀质量学习的文化。如果没有分析根本原因，就有可能把改进工作的重点放在错误的问题上。例如，当问题不在于员工的技能，而在于他们没有时间做完所有的事情时，对员工进行再培训。理想情况下，应尽可能避免抱怨，积极寻求对患者和工作人员有效或无效的反馈。

用户研究

用户研究在简单的反馈之上，有助于了解所服务的用户情况，如他们的体验、需求、行为和动机。用户研究可以为设计更好的用户服务提供有价值的见解。在医疗保健领域，用户包括患者和护理人员。但是，在考虑改进服务时，也包括将患者转诊或转出服务机

service, they may also include other professionals who are referring in to your service and those services you refer patients on to, as they are also users of the information you provide. You can learn about users and their needs through a variety of methods, including accessing research reports, conducting interviews, observing them while using your service and talking to other people who work closely with your patients (such as carers and advocacy workers).

The challenge of value

Over recent years there has been an increasing focus in healthcare on the concept of value, which can be defined as delivering the best possible outcomes at both the individual patient and population level, at the lowest possible cost. See Chapter 1 for a more detailed discussion of this 'triple aim'. Assessing value requires a much greater focus on population health and understanding what outcomes matter for an individual patient. These are likely to include a mixture of clinical outcomes and patient reported outcome (or experience) measures or PROMS (or PREMS) (Devlin and Appleby, 2010) which often include data around mental, physical and social functioning (Box 6.2).

Assessing the extent to which your team or service is delivering value also requires an understanding that value can be negatively impacted by both the under and overuse of healthcare. An example of work focused on reducing the overuse of healthcare is the Choosing Wisely campaign in the UK, led by the Academy of Medical Royal Colleges (www. choosingwisely.co.uk).

构的专业人员，因为他们也是为你提供信息的用户。可以通过各种方法了解用户及其需求，包括分析研究报告、做访谈、在提供服务时观察用户以及与患者密切合作的人（如护理人员和宣传工作者）交谈。

价值的挑战

近年来，医学界越来越关注价值的概念，价值可以定义为以尽可能低的成本在患者和更广泛的人群提供尽可能好的结果。有关"三重目标"更详细的讨论，参见第 1 章。评估价值需要更多地关注公民健康，了解结果对患者的重要性。这些可能包括临床结果和患者报告结果（或体验）测量（PROMS 或 PREMS）（Devlin 和 Appleby，2010 年），其中通常包括有关精神、身体和社会功能的数据（框 6.2）。

评估团队或服务机构在多大程度上提供了价值，还需要了解医疗保健缺乏和过度使用会对价值产生负面影响。英国皇家医学院（Academy of Medical Royal Colleges）领导的"明智选择"（Choosing Wisely）运动就是一个致力于减少过度医疗的例子 (www. choosingwisely.co.uk)。

Box 6.2 From 'what's the matter with you' to 'what matters to you?'
框 6.2   从"你怎么了"到"什么对你最重要？"

Finding out more about what your patients want from your service can inform both individual care plans and wider service redesign. The 'What Matters to You' movement is a practical example of doing this in practice. It encourages clinicians to ask patients what matters to them on the basis that, as well as helping to establish a relationship, it provides you with crucial insights that mean you are able to tailor care to deliver the best possible outcomes for that individual patient. See www.whatmatterstoyou.scot for further information.

尽可能了解患者对服务的需求可以为个人护理计划和更广泛的服务设计提供信息。"什么对你最重要"运动是实践的一个实例。它鼓励临床医生询问患者对他们来说什么重要，因为它不仅有助于建立关系，还提供了重要的见解，这意味着能够定制护理服务，尽可能为患者提供最佳结果。更多信息参见 www.whatmatterstoyou.scot。

Given that the time available to do improvement work is limited and that most services have multiple issues they could focus on, thinking about where you are likely to have the largest impact on 'value' can help in making the important decision of what to focus on first.

考虑到可用于改进工作的时间有限，而且大多数服务机构都有多个需要关注的问题，思考对"价值"产生最大影响的地方，有助于做出首先应关注什么的重要决策。

Anticipating problems before they happen

在问题发生之前预见问题

Ideally a team or service needs to build in ongoing mechanisms for monitoring whether it is meeting key quality standards. This is known as quality control (see Chapter 1) and is part of a comprehensive approach to managing the quality of care. But this doesn't mean you need to measure everything all of the time. Some indicators will be routinely measured as part of your electronic clinical records and in these situations the IT system can be set up to provide an alert if a standard slips. Where data is not routinely collected, you can use routine sampling to check performance against key standards. Ideally, you also want to find ways to encourage patients and their families to routinely feed back on key quality issues so that they become an active part of your system for monitoring the quality of your service.

理想情况下，团队或服务机构需要建立持续的机制来监视其是否符合关键的质量标准。这就是所谓的质量控制（请参阅第 1 章），是管理护理质量的综合方法的一部分。但这并不意味着需要一直测量所有内容。仅将电子临床记录的一部分指标进行常规测量，在这些情况下，可以设置 IT 系统以在指标不合格时提供警报。如果不定期收集数据，则可以使用常规采样来对照关键标准检查绩效。理想情况下，还希望找到鼓励患者及其家人定期反馈关键质量问题的方法，他们积极的反溃可以监控服务质量。

References
参考文献

Devlin N and Appleby J. (2010) *Getting the Most Out Of PROMS*, London, The Kings Fund.

Powell AE, Davies HTO and Thomson RG. (2003) Using routine comparative data to assess the quality of health care: understanding and avoiding common pitfalls *BMJ Quality & Safety*, 121, 22-128.

Pringle M, Bradley CP, Carmichael CM et al. (1995). Significant event auditing. A study of the feasibility and potential of casebased auditing in primary medical care. *Occasional Paper Royal College of General Practitioners*, 70, i-viii, 1-71.

Further reading and resources
深度阅读与资源

National Clinical Audits:

- The Healthcare Quality Improvement Partnership (HQIP) is an independent organisation led by the Academy of Medical Royal Colleges, The Royal College of Nursing and National Voices. HQIP commissions, manages, supports and promotes national and local programmes of quality improvement. This includes the National and Local clinical audit programmes, the Clinical Outcome Review Programmes and the National Joint Registry on behalf of NHS England and other healthcare departments and organisations. www. hqip.org.uk.

- In Northern Ireland, the Regulation and Quality Improvement Authority (RQIA) conducts a programme of clinical audits of health and social care services. www. rqia.org.uk/what-we-do/rqia-s-funding-programme/rqia-clinical-audit-programme/.
- Scottish Healthcare Audits maintains a wide range of national clinical audits, many of which are specialitybased and involve a wide range of clinical, government and voluntary sector stakeholders. www. isdscotland.org/Health-Topics/Scottish-Healthcare-Audits.
- The NHS Wales programme of audits includes the majority of the NCAPOP audits as well as a number of other national or multiorganisational audits recognised by the National Clinical Audit and Outcome Review Advisory Committee. www.gov.wales/topics/health/publications/ health/reports/clinical-audit/?lang=en.

Chapter 7

Understanding the Problem

第 7 章 理解问题

Joanna Bircher

General Practitioner, Lockside Medical Centre, Stalybridge, UK
Clinical Director of Greater Manchester GP Excellence Programme, Manchester, UK
Quality Improvement Clinical Lead for Tameside and Glossop Clinical Commissioning Group, Tameside, UK

OVERVIEW
概述

- After an area has been identified for improvement, it is helpful to explore the problem in more detail before planning and implementing changes.
  在确定了需要改进的领域之后，可以在规划和实施变革之前更详细地探讨问题。
- A variety of tools and methods have been shown to be useful.
  一系列有用的工具和方法。
- Choose the tool depending on the type of issue identified for improvement.
  根据改进问题的类型选择工具。
- Involving patients and team members will help achieve a better understanding of the problem.
  让患者和团队成员参与有助于更好地理解问题。

Chapter 6 described how to identify areas of work that could be improved, and how to prioritise these. Once the subject for the quality improvement activity has been selected, it is tempting to leap in to start 'fixing' things. If you do this without a full enough understanding of the problem, you may choose interventions that are less likely to lead to sustainable improvement. Quality improvement is best viewed as a team sport, and the chance a project will be successful is increased when all those involved have a shared understanding of the issues. This chapter explores techniques you can use to gain a deeper understanding of the issue prior to planning and testing out your interventions to implement change. Methods for understanding the problem fall into two broad categories:

- Methods that look more deeply into the factors that are resulting in poor performance or outcomes. This process is called 'root

第 6 章描述了如何确定改进的工作领域，以及如何确定这些领域的优先级。一旦选择了质量改进的主题，就很有可能跳进去"修复"一些事情。如果你在没有充分理解问题的情况下这样做，则可能会选择不太可能导致可持续改进的干预措施。质量改进最好被视为一项团队运动，当所有相关人员都对问题有共同的理解时，项目成功的机会就会增加。本章探讨在规划和测试实施变革的干预措施之前，可以使用哪些技术来加深对问题的理解。理解问题的方法分为两大类：

- 更深入地研究导致不良绩效或结果的因素，这个过程叫做"根本原因分析"。有用的工具包括"5 个为什么""鱼骨图或石川图"。

cause analysis'. Useful tools include the Five Whys and Fishbone or Ishikawa diagrams.

- Methods to gain a broader perspective on an existing service or process in order to identify change ideas, or to encourage teams to build on good work that is already happening. Tools in this category include process mapping and appreciative inquiry.

Gaining a deeper, or broader, understanding of your problem area makes it easier to plan and test out your changes. You can then use what you have learned through these activities to construct a driver diagram, which will clarify how you believe your change ideas will lead to the improvement you want to see. A driver diagram can also readily be turned into a 'plan on a page' for your quality improvement activity.

Tools to explore causal factors

5 Whys

The 5 Whys technique was originally developed by Sakichi Toyota and was used within the Toyota Motor Corporation during the evolution of its manufacturing methodologies (Ohno, 1988). The simple act of asking 'why' in a structured participative way can uncover important factors related to human behaviour and our working environment that contribute either to poor performance or inefficient processes and systems. The method involves repeatedly asking the question 'why' (five is an arbitrary but useful target). Each answer will lead you to another question until you get to the root cause of the problem. Although this technique is called 5 Whys you may find that you will need to ask the question fewer, or more, times than five before you get to the issue at the heart of the problem. The example in Box 7.1 explores why waiting times are so long in the outpatient department.

This technique not only helps identify the root cause of a problem but also the relationship between different root causes of a problem. Its simplicity is attractive as it is easy to complete without statistical analysis. It is a particularly useful technique when problems involve human factors or interactions and when there are simple, linear reasons behind a problem. It is less helpful to explore complex, multifactorial problems. In this situation, the 5 Whys approach can be expanded and structure in the form of a Fishbone diagram.

- 可以从更广泛的角度对现有服务或流程进行观察，从而确定变革思路，或鼓励团队利用已经应用的良好工作方法。此类别中的工具包括过程映射和肯定式探询。

对问题领域有了更深入或更广泛的了解，就更容易计划和测试变革方案。然后，可以使用通过这些活动所学到的知识来构建驱动图，该图将阐明变革思路如何导致希望看到的改进。驱动图也可以很容易地变成"计划表"，以进行质量改进活动。

探索起因的工具

"5 个为什么"

"5 个为什么"最初是由丰田佐吉开发的，并在丰田汽车公司的制造方法演变过程中使用（Ohno，1988 年）。以结构化的参与方式问"为什么"的简单行为可以发现与人类行为和工作环境相关的重要因素，这些因素会导致绩效不佳或流程和系统效率低下。这个方法包括反复问"为什么"（"5"是一个任意但有用的目标）。每一个答案都会引出另一个问题，直到找到问题的根本原因。尽管这一技巧被称为"5 个为什么"，但你可能会发现，在进入问题的核心之前，需要问的问题可能比 5 个少，也许会更多。框 7.1 中的示例探讨了门诊部等待时间如此之长的原因。

该方法不仅有助于确定问题的根本原因，还可以帮助确定多个根本原因之间的关系。它因简单而吸引人，因为无需统计分析即可轻松完成。当问题涉及人为因素或相互作用，并且问题背后有简单的线性原因时，这是一种特别有用的技术。但对于探索复杂的多因素问题没有太大帮助，在这种情况下，"5 个为什么"方法可以扩展，并以鱼骨图的形式构建。

Box 7.1 **Example of a 5 Whys exercise.**

框 7.1 **"5 个为什么"练习示例**

Problem Statement:

问题陈述：

The waiting time in the outpatient department is on average 40–60 minutes.

门诊的等候时间平均为 40~60 分钟。

1 Why are patients waiting so long?

为什么患者要等这么久？

- Because the consultant doesn't start the clinic until 40 minutes after the first appointment slot.

  因为会诊医生在第 1 次预约时间后 40 分钟才来到诊所。

2 Why does the consultant arrive late?

会诊医生为什么迟到？

- Because the management meeting is scheduled for the hour before the clinic and it always runs over time.

  因为管理会议是在开诊前 1 小时安排的，而且总是超时。

3 Why does the management meeting run over time?

为什么管理会议超时？

- Because the agenda is too full for the time allocated.

  因为议程太满了。

4 Why is the agenda too full for the time allocated?

为什么议程太满？

- Because anyone can add anything to the agenda.

  因为任何人都可以在议程上添加内容。

5 Why can anyone add anything to the agenda?

为什么任何人都可以在议程上添加内容？

- Because no one has been asked to co-ordinate the agenda, prioritise items or allocate time.

  因为没有人要求协调议程、安排优先事项或分配时间。

Fishbone diagram

Getting a team to create a fishbone (Ishikawa, or cause and effect) diagram (Ishikawa, 1968) helps to generate a shared understanding of a problem, when multiple factors may be contributing. It helps to ensure important potential factors are not ignored and at the same time sorts ideas into useful categories.

To create a fishbone diagram, first identify the problem, which becomes the head of the fish. Then, ask the group to think of the main categories of causes of the problem – in the example shown these are environment, organisation, clinicians and patients; these form the spines of the fish. Discuss each major category, adding the ideas generated as sub-branches. Each sub-branch may be further broken down into its contributing factors. For every spine and sub-branch identified, ask 'Why

鱼骨图

让团队创建鱼骨图（又称石川图或因果图）（Ishikawa，1968 年）有助于在多个因素可能起作用的情况下形成对问题的共同理解。它有助于确保重要的潜在因素不被忽视，同时将想法分类为有用的类别。

要创建鱼骨图，首先确定问题所在，问题所在就是鱼头。然后，让小组思考问题原因的主要类别——在示例中，这些类别是环境、组织、临床医生和患者，它们形成了鱼的刺。讨论每个主要类别，将产生的想法添加为子分支。每个子分支可进一步细分为其影响因素。对于确定的每个脊椎和子分支，追问"为什么会发生这种情况？"并从不同

does this happen?' and consider the question from different perspectives; in our example, these might be patient, administrator, nurse, doctor and commissioner. This will produce the layers of causes that will help you to fully understand the root of the problem and its dependencies. Use your completed diagram to help you generate ideas for improvement.

The Fishbone diagram in Figure 7.1 was created to help a practice team understand why so many of their patients with asthma had failed to attend for the recommended annual review with the nurse.

Tools to gain a broader perspective

Process mapping

Our day-to-day work in healthcare includes a wide range of processes that ensure safe and effective delivery of care for patients. Examples of such processes include the management of repeat prescriptions, the handling of investigation results and the experience of a patient through an outpatient department. There is a possibility of error at every stage, and errors can lead to harm to patient; though more often, they lead to inefficiencies and wasted time. Poor processes may, for instance, result in a patient spending hours in a waiting room, only to find once they see the doctor that the results that they came for can't be accessed.

Changing inefficient processes, especially those that are long established, can be complex and difficult. For improvement activities to be effective the first step is for all those involved to fully understand the existing process, including steps they may not be involved in. Process mapping generates this understanding by creating a visual representation. This is created as follows:

- The facilitator explains process mapping to the participants, making it clear that each step needs to be broken down – the more detailed the better – because this will help identify inefficiencies in the process and potential waste.
- The start and end point of the process are defined. For repeat prescribing, the start point could be the patient requesting a repeat prescription. The end point could be the patient collecting the prescription.

角度考虑问题。在这个例子中，这可能是患者、管理人员、护士、医生和专员。这将产生一系列原因，帮助充分理解问题的根源及其分支，图表能够帮助产生改进的思路。

图 7.1 中的鱼骨图是为了帮助工作团队理解为什么许多哮喘患者没有参加护士推荐的年度评估。

获得更广阔视角的工具

流程映射

我们在医疗保健领域的日常工作包括为患者提供一系列安全有效的护理流程。此类流程包括重复处方的管理、调查结果的处理以及患者在门诊的体验。每一个阶段都有出错的可能，出错会对患者造成伤害，虽然更多的时候会导致效率低下和浪费时间。例如，糟糕的流程可能会导致患者在候诊室待上数小时，结果在看医生后发现无法获取他们想要的结果。

改变低效的流程复杂而困难，尤其是那些已经建立很久的流程。为了使改进有效，第一步是让所有相关人员充分了解现有流程，包括他们不参与的步骤。流程映射通过创建一个可视化图表来理解。创建如下：

- 主持人向参与者解释流程映射，明确指出每个步骤都需要分解，越详细越好——因为这将有助于识别流程中的低效和潜在的浪费。
- 确定流程的起点和终点。对于重复开处方，起始点可以是患者请求给予上次的处方，终点是患者领取处方。

Step 1
步骤 1

Steps 3 and 4
步骤 3 和步骤 4

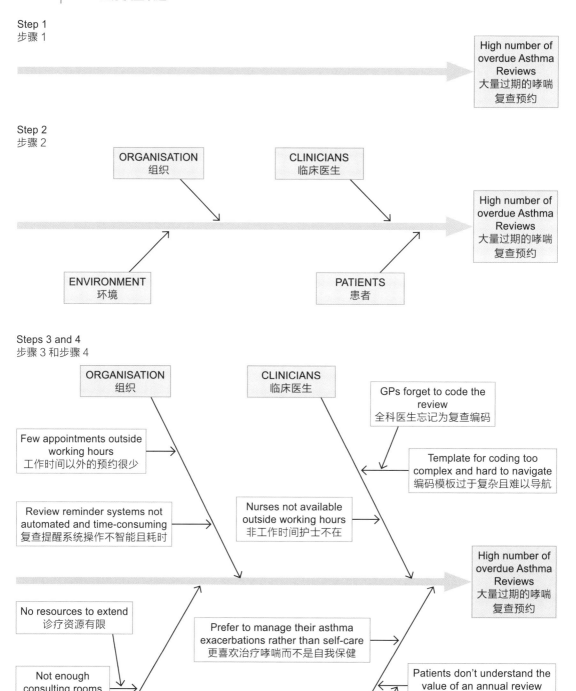

Figure 7.1 Example of a Fishbone diagram.

图 7.1 鱼骨图示例

- If one step can be done in several ways, this is added vertically; for example, in the repeat prescribing process the patient may request a script in different ways.
- Once the map is created, the facilitator asks the group where the problems arise. The participants then note the problems on a differently coloured sticky notes and attach these at the appropriate point on the map.
- Participants are then asked to identify possible solutions to test out. These are noted on another different coloured sticky note. They are stuck over the problems that were identified.

Process mapping often highlights that the more steps there are in a process, the more likely it is there is inefficiency. It is a good idea to leave the map on display for a few weeks so that any issues that arise during implementation can be more easily discussed. Once the solutions have been tested out and implemented, it can be helpful to reconvene the group to recreate the new process, with the problem areas sorted and waste minimised. Ask the group: is the new process working in the way predicted? Are there any new problems, or have any unintended steps been created?

The example process map in Figure 7.2 has been used to identify the various steps involved in repeat prescribing at a GP practice.

Appreciative Inquiry

The methods described so far have focused on achieving an understanding of problems that occur during the delivery of care for patients. It can also be helpful to understand more fully what goes well and appreciative inquiry is a technique that enables this (Lewis et al., 2011) (Box 7.2). It is an approach to improvement that shifts the focus from 'What is wrong with our service and how can we fix it?' to 'What is going well and how can we build on this?' Building on 'what's strong, not what's wrong' can have a positive influence on the culture of an organisation. It can be especially helpful to improve morale when working in difficult circumstances and create a culture that is more conducive to quality improvement.

It is your choice whether to use a structured appreciative inquiry process, or whether to just become more appreciative in general when approaching improvement. For example, when

- 如果一个步骤可以通过多种方式完成，则垂直添加。例如，在重复开处方的流程中，患者可以以不同的方式请求脚本。
- 创建映射图后，主持人会询问小组问题出现的位置。然后，参与者在不同颜色的便签上记下问题，并将其贴在映射图的适当位置。
- 然后要求参与者找出可能的解决方案并进行测试。另一张不同颜色的便笺上注明了这些内容。他们对发现的问题束手无策。

流程映射常常强调，流程中的步骤越多，效率就越低。最好将映射图保留几周，以便讨论实现过程中出现的所有问题。一旦找到解决方案并实施，需重新召集小组创建新的流程，将问题分类并将浪费最小化。要询问小组：新流程是否能按照预期的方式工作？是否产生了新问题或意外的步骤？

图 7.2 中的示例流程图描述了全科医生重复开处方所涉及的各个步骤

肯定式探询

到目前为止所描述的方法都集中在理解为患者提供护理过程中出现的问题上。对于更全面地了解哪些事件进展顺利也很有帮助，而肯定式探询是一种实现这一点的技术（Lewis 等，2011 年）（框 7.2）。这是一种改进方法，它将重点从"我们的服务有什么问题，我们如何解决？"转移到"哪些事件进展顺利，在此基础上如何发展？"建立在"什么是强大的，而不是什么是错误的"的基础上，可以对组织的文化产生积极的影响。在困难的环境下工作，尤其有助于提高士气，创造有利于提高质量的文化。

可以选择使用结构化的肯定式探询过程，也可以在接近改进时总体上再开始比较肯定式的探询。例如，在团队会议上查看患者调

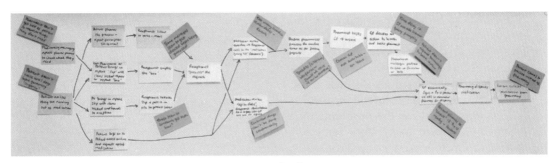

Figure 7.2 Example of process map.
图 7.2   流程图示例

Box 7.2 Appreciative Inquiry – the 5 Ds.
框 7.2   肯定式探询——5 个 D

Define the area you want to focus on.
定义（Define）要关注的领域。

Discover the positive stories relate to the area of focus. Explore the experience of the clinicians, managers, administrators and patients using positively framed open questions such as 'What do you like best about …?' and then taking the inquiry to a deeper level 'Why does that work well for you?' The language used in your inquiry is critical to whether the inquiry generates further positive change.
发现（Discover）与重点领域有关的积极故事。使用积极性的开放式问题探索临床医生、经理、管理人员和患者的体验，例如"你最喜欢……什么？"，然后将询问深入到"为什么这对你有用？"调查中使用的语言对调查是否可以产生进一步的积极变化至关重要。

Discover the stories that most reflect the high points, those that seem to be most inspiring and generate a sense of optimism. The leader collates the key features in the stories and presents them back to the team.
找出（Discover）最能反映高光时刻的故事，那些似乎最能鼓舞人心、产生乐观情绪的故事。领导者要整理故事中的关键特征，并将它们呈现给团队。

Dream. The positive energy generated is then used to imagine a future service, where the high points discovered become part of everyday reality.
梦想（Dream）。产生的正能量被用来设想未来，这种状态将成为日常生活的一部分。

Design. This final step puts the details on any changes agreed to move the team or organisation towards their 'dream'. If the approach is to make a sustainable difference, then it is important to notice and celebrate successes that are contributing towards achieving the dream.
设计（Design）。最后一步将详细说明任何能够将团队或组织推向他们"梦想"的变革。如果这种方法是为了实现可持续的改变，那么就等着庆祝梦想实现吧。

---

reviewing patient survey results at your team meeting you could decide to start by highlighting what the patients like best about your service.

Driver diagrams

So far we have looked at tools and techniques that aim to achieve a shared, deeper level understanding of areas for improvement. These activities can generate such a wealth of change ideas it can feel overwhelming. It is easy to lose sight of the overall aim, and how each change

查结果时，您可以从强调患者最喜欢的服务开始。

驱动图

到目前为止，我们已经研究了旨在实现对改进领域做更深入共享的工具和方法。这些活动可以产生如此丰富的变革理念，让人感觉势不可挡。我们很容易忽视整体目标，

is designed to drive the improvement you are aiming for. A driver diagram is a tool to help organise and display planned improvements in a logical way – to clearly explain your 'theory of change'. The diagram is focused around a single clear improvement aim, though some organisations will use a driver diagram to plan the direction of their work following development of a vision or mission statement. A useful driver diagram can only be created once you have a achieved a detailed understanding of the problem you are trying to solve by using the tools/methods already described.

There are typically four levels to a driver diagram:

- The aim is what you are trying to achieve, and ideally is something measurable. A well - worded aim makes it easy to define what will be measured.
- The primary drivers are an agreed set of broad areas that influence your aim; essentially the areas that require work or improvement.
- The secondary drivers are the more specific influences that shape your primary drivers. Each primary driver will be influenced by several secondary drivers. Secondary drivers may impact on more than one primary driver.
- Change ideas are generated by the work you have already done as a team to fully understand the problem that needs to be fixed and are ideas that your team would like to test. A change idea should affect at least one secondary driver and each change idea should, of course, contribute to achieving the aim.

When completed, the driver diagram provides a clearly portrayed change strategy that can be shared and provide the basis for planning the individual projects or interventions. The diagram should not be considered 'fixed' and can change over time as improvements are generated. The example in Figure 7.3 relates to a primary care 'walk-in centre' with a high rate of antibiotic prescribing when compared to similar centres. The team constructed a driver diagram having explored the issues that were contributing to the high prescribing.

只关注如何设计每一个变革行动来推动所追求的改进目标。驱动图是一种工具，能清楚地解释你的"变革理论"，可以帮助组织有逻辑的梳理改进计划。该图的重点在于所围绕的明确的改进目标，有些组织会在制定愿景或使命后使用驱动图来规划其工作方向。只有在通过使用前面描述的工具和方法对试图解决的问题有了详细了解之后，才能创建有用的驱动图。

驱动图通常有 4 个级别：

- 目标，即正在努力实现的目标，理想情况下是可以测量的。用词准确的目标使我们很容易定义将要测量的内容。
- 主要驱动因素，是指影响目标的一系列广泛因素，基本上是需要改进的领域。
- 次要驱动因素以更具体的形式塑造主要驱动因素。每个主要驱动因素都会受到几个次要驱动因素的影响，次要驱动因素可能会影响多个主要驱动因素。
- 变革理念是团队在已经完成的工作中产生的，以充分理解需要解决的问题，并且是团队希望测试的想法。一个变革的想法应该至少影响一个次要驱动因素，当然，每个变革的想法都应该有助于实现目标。

完成后，驱动图提供了一个清晰描述的变革策略，可以共享，并为规划单个项目或干预提供基础。驱动图不应该是固定的，应该可以随着时间的推移而改变。图 7.3 中的示例与初级保健"随到随诊中心"有关，与类似中心相比，该中心的抗生素处方率较高。该团队构建了一个驱动图，探讨了导致高处方率的问题。

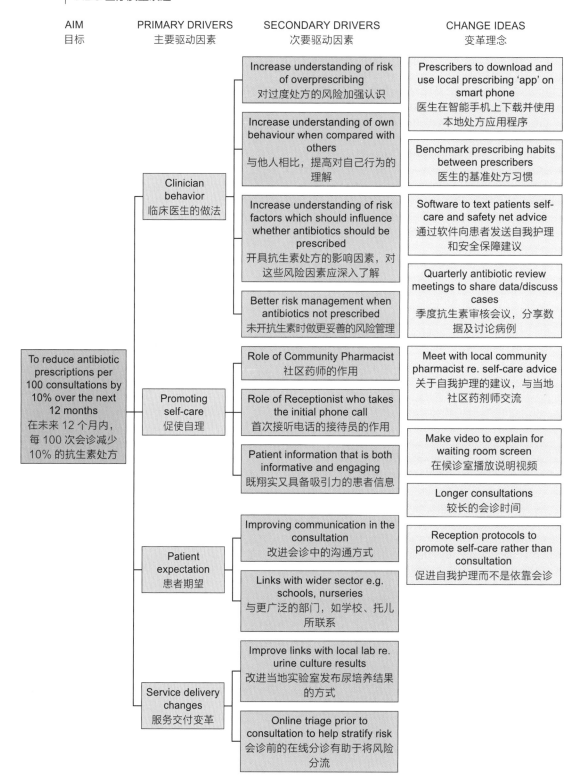

Figure 7.3 Example of a driver diagram.

图 7.3 驱动图示例

Conclusion

There are many tools available to help you explore the identified problem or issue in more detail (see Further reading) but those described in this chapter are the most frequently deployed. Choosing and using the right tool will ensure that your quality improvement activity is addressed at the right part of the system. The processes involved are also invaluable for getting staff and patients on board and securing engagement with your project. Both are prerequisites for success.

结论

有许多工具可以更深入地探索已识别的问题（请参阅深度阅读），但本章中描述的工具是最常用的。选择和使用正确的工具，将确保质量改进在系统的正确部分得以进行。对于确保员工和患者参与项目，所涉及的流程是非常宝贵的，两者都是成功的先决条件。

References
参考文献

Ishikawa K. (1968) *Guide to Quality Control*, Tokyo, JUSE.

Lewis S, Passmore J and Cantore S. (2011) *Appreciative Inquiry for Change Management: Using AI to Facilitate Organizational Development*, London, Kogan-Page.

Ohno T. (1988) *Toyota Production System: Beyond Large-scale Production*, Portland, OR, Productivity Press.

Further reading and resources
深度阅读与相关资源

Gillam S and Siriwardena AN. (2014) *Quality Improvement in Primary Care: The Essential Guide*, Oxford, Radcliffe.

Langley G, Moen R, Nolan K et al. (2009) *The Improvement Guide: A Practical Approach to Enhancing Organizational Performance*, San Francisco, CA, Jossey-Bass.

A suite of free resources from the Institute of Healthcare Improvement to support improvement and the management of change: www.ihi.org/resources/Pages/HowtoImprove.

A collection of tools and guidance to support quality improvement activities in the primary care setting from the Royal College of General Practitioners: www.rcgp.org.uk/clinical-and-research/our-programmes/quality-improvement.aspx.

A brief introduction, from the Health Foundation, to some common approaches used to improve quality, their underlying principles, effectiveness and applicability within the healthcare arena: www.health.org.uk/publications/quality-improvement-made-simple.

Improvement ideas, tools and resources from across the health sector presented in a searchable online 'hub' from NHS Improvement, designed to facilitate collaboration and sharing: https://improvement.nhs.uk/resources.

第 8 章 | 开发和测试解决方案

James Mountford

Director of Quality, Royal Free London NHS Foundation Trust, London, UK Editor in Chief, BMJ Leader, London, UK

OVERVIEW
概述

- Solutions need to be developed, prioritised and tested, as changes which in theory seem likely to result in improvement, may in practice turn out to be ineffective.
  解决方案需要开发、确定优先次序并进行测试，否则从理论上看可能会导致改进的变革，在实践中失效。

- Various tools and techniques are used to develop solutions. The process starts with divergent thinking to generate ideas, then convergent thinking to prioritise those ideas and take them through to testing.
  有各种工具和技术用于开发解决方案。这个过程从发散思维产生想法开始，然后用聚合性思维为这些想法确定优先次序，并对其测试。

- Testing in improvement depends on cycles of learning, with results of previous cycles informing what is next tested. Each test is underpinned by a theory and prediction about what will happen; actual results are compared to those predicted.
  改进测试取决于学习周期，前一个周期的结果会告知下一步要测试的内容。每个测试都以理论和对即将发生的事情的预测为基础，将实际结果与预测的结果进行比较。

- Various models can be used to test solutions and one of the best known in healthcare is the Plan Do Study Act (PDSA) cycle.
  有各种模式可用于测试解决方案,其中在医疗领域最著名的是"计划－执行－研究－行动"（PDSA）循环。

- Tests should start out small scale and results critically reviewed. 'Adopt, adapt or abandon' is a useful maxim.
  测试应从小规模开始，并严格审查结果。"采用、修改或放弃"是很有用的准则。

- The best way to assess a well-formed plan is to test it in a real-life context in a controlled way, repeatedly measuring what matters.
  评估一个设计良好的计划的最佳方法，是在现实环境中以可控的方式对其进行测试，反复测量重要的事情。

Why develop and test solutions?

为什么要开发和测试解决方案？

Previous chapters have described how to determine what to improve, how to develop a solid understanding of the problem and have recommended tools for doing this efficiently and robustly. Without a grounding in improvement, our instinctive solution to the problem may

前面的章节介绍了如何确定要改进的方面，如何对问题有扎实的理解，并推荐了有效而稳健的工具。如果没有改进的基础，我们对问题的本能解决方案可能是建议"增加

be to suggest 'more of the same' – more time, more equipment, more people. But improvement should usually involve accomplishing better results with the resources that are available (or even with less resource). Another issue is the assumption that bright, knowledgeable, hard-working and well-intentioned people, expert in the area, 'know' what will work best. This can lead to changes being implemented at scale and only then discovering that the changes do not work as expected,that they have unintended consequences or that they may even be making things worse. A related issue is 'planning paralysis' where teams refine seemingly sensible solutions in committee, only to find that when a change hits reality in implementation, it does not work as expected. This reminds us not to let the perfect be the enemy of the good – better is most often built in a series of linked steps and learning cycles (Gawande, 2008).

Mindful of these pitfalls, the Sheffield geriatrician Tom Downes has coined the phrase 'great care is discovered, not decided' highlighting the importance of developing and testing solutions in structured, controlled ways, linked to the measurement of outcome, process and balancing metrics and resources used.

Improvement also highlights (and can fill) a gap in traditional ways of knowing. Traditionally, doctors have been trained to think that knowledge comes from evidence published in journals and one's own anecdotal experience. Improvement focuses on an important additional way of knowing: 'what works in my context' – translating the evidence base into the care patients actually receive, every time. Measurement is the focus of the next chapter. This chapter focuses on how to develop and test changes in an efficient, effective and creative way.

Developing solutions

We saw in Chapter 7 how various tools are used to refine our understanding of the problem under scrutiny and ways to understand the system. Improvement methods focus on changing the system which produces the outcome we are working on either by: (i) making incremental changes to the current system; or (ii) by changing the system in a fundamental way. These are sometimes called, respectively,

更多东西"——更多的时间、更多的设备、更多的人。但是改进通常应该包括用可用的资源（甚至更少的资源）取得更好的结果。另一个问题是，假设该领域中聪明、知识渊博、工作努力、心地善良的专家知道什么最有效。这可能导致大规模地实施变革，然后才发现变革未按预期工作，产生了意想不到的后果，甚至可能使情况变得更糟。一个相关的问题是"计划瘫痪"，团队对委员会审核中看似合理的解决方案精益求精，却发现当一个变革在实施中触及现实时，并没有如预期那样起作用。这提醒我们不要让完美成为"良好"的敌人——"良好"往往建立在一系列相互联系的步骤和学习周期中（Gawande，2008 年）。

考虑到这些陷阱，谢菲尔德的老年医学专家汤姆·唐斯创造了"伟大的护理是被发现的，而不是被决定的"这一格言，强调了以结构化、可控的方式开发和测试解决方案的重要性，该方法与结果、过程的测量相联系，并平衡所使用的指标和资源。

改进还突出显示了（并可以填补）传统认识方式的空白。传统上，经过训练医生认为知识来自发表在期刊上的证据和自己的轶事经历。改进聚焦于另外一种重要的认知方式："在我的环境中什么是有效的"——将证据基础转化为患者每次实际接受的护理。测量是下一章的重点，本章重点介绍如何以高效、有效和创造性的方式开展和测试变革。

开发解决方案

在第 7 章中，我们详细了解了如何使用各种工具来加深对问题的理解以及了解系统的工作方式。改进方法的重点是通过以下方式改变我们为之奋斗的系统：对当前系统进行渐进性变革，或从根本上变革系统。有时分别将它们称为"反应性"或类型 1 变革，

'reactive' or Type 1, and 'fundamental' or Type 2 changes. In either case, the focus is on changing how routine work gets done – in other words, the inputs and standard processes followed. The Improvement Guide (Langley, et al., 2009) identifies three basic approaches to developing a change which results in improvement:

- From clear understanding of processes and systems ofwork.
- From adapting known good ideas.
- From creative thinking.

In the early stages of developing solutions, teams should use their diversity to generate ideas (divergent thinking) stemming from (for example) their process mapping, fishbone analyses and driver diagrams.

Ideas then need to be prioritised to determine which ideas to test, and in what order (convergent thinking). Tools and techniques are available for each, which include the following:

Generating ideas

In this phase, the objective is to generate as many ideas as possible, without evaluating them.

- Brainstorming: Here, team members (either in rotation or randomly) contribute ideas which are noted by a facilitator. This method is simple, rapid and often fun.
- Nominal group technique: This is a 'silent brainstorm',whereby team members write down ideas in silence. The key advantage over brainstorming is encouraging contributions from introverted team members and flattening hierarchies.

Box 8.1 provides a worked example of the sort of outputs that might be expected from an idea-generation exercise for falls reduction in hospitals.

Prioritising ideas

- *Multi-voting:* Here, each team member gets a certain number of votes (typically 5–8) which they can allocate to the range of ideas under scrutiny. Different versions include a requirement only to vote once for each idea, or free allocation (where someone can put all their votes on one option if they wish). This method is most effective when there are a larger (8 or more) number of options. Votes are tallied and options with the greatest

以及"二本"或类型 2 变革。无论哪种情况，重点都在于变革常规工作的完成方式，换句话说，就是遵循规范的输入和标准流程。《改进指南》（Langley 等，2009 年）确定了 3 种基本方法，来开展能够导致改进的变革：

- 对工作流程和系统的清晰理解。
- 调整已有的好想法。
- 创造性思维。

在开发解决方案的早期阶段，团队应该利用他们的多样性，从（例如）流程图、鱼骨分析和驱动图中产生想法（发散思维）。

然后需要对想法进行优先排序，以确定测试哪些想法，以及测试顺序（聚合思维）。工具和技术适用于每种类型，包括：

产生想法

在这个阶段，目标是产生尽可能多的想法，而不是评估它们。

- 头脑风暴：在这里，团队成员（轮流或随机）提出建议，并由主持人记录。这种方法简单、快速，而且常常很有趣。
- 名义群体法：这是一个"无声的头脑风暴"，团队成员在沉默中写下想法。与头脑风暴相比，关键的优势在于鼓励内向的团队成员发挥技能，并使层次结构扁平化。

框 8.1 提供了 1 个工作示例，说明了减少医院内跌倒的创意生成练习可能会产生的输出结果。

为想法排序

- 多次投票：每个团队成员都有一定数量的票（通常为 5~8 票），他们可以将这些票投给正在审查的各种想法。每个想法的不同版本只能投票 1 次，或者自由投票（如果愿意，某人可以将所有投票都放在 1 个选项上）。当选项数量较大（8 个或更多）时，此方法最

Box 8.1 **Example: Developing ideas to test to reduce falls in hospital wards.**
框 8.1　**示例：开发测试想法以减少医院病房的跌倒**

From clear understanding of ward environment, processes and systems of work
对病房环境、流程和工作系统的清晰认识

Staffing
人员配备

- levels
  水平档次。
- skill mix
  技能混合。
- use of 1:1 care (specialing).
  使用 1：1 护理（专业化）。

Physical environment
物理环境

- furniture
  家具。
- lighting
  灯光。
- trip hazards
  障碍物。
- floor material
  地板材料。
- rails and handles in toilets and bathrooms.
  厕所和浴室的栏杆和把手。

Ward activities
病房活动

- daily activities
  日常活动。
- mobilization
  转移。
- therapist input
  治疗师给予支持。

Clothing: fit and comfort.
服装：舒适

From taking and adapting known good ideas
采用和调整已有的好想法

Communication, education and training:
交流、教育和培训：

- raise awareness of fall prevalence, harm and potential to improve, e.g. at staff meetings, through posters, newsletters, WhatsApp groups
  通过海报、时事通讯、在线小组等方式，提高对跌倒率、危害和改善潜力的认识。
- manual handling procedures and support.
  手动处理程序和支持设备。

Identifying risk factors:
识别风险因素：

- risk assessments.
  风险评估。

- physical health needs: hydration, continence
  身体健康需求：补水、节制。
- confusion and mental health factors.
  精神困扰和心理健康因素。
- medication review and substitution.
  药物检查和替代。

'Everything I need to hand':
"我需要处理的一切"：

- declutter patient areas, personal items visible and accessible.
  整理患者区域，可见、可触及的个人物品。
- call-bell readily available.
  随时可用的呼叫铃。

Individualised care plans
个性化护理计划

Falls packs available in toilet/bathroom to avoid staff leaving patient to get materials needed.
厕所／浴室提供防摔背包，以避免工作人员离开患者去获取所需的材料。

Non-slip socks and shoes.
防滑袜子、鞋。

From creative thinking
创造性思维

Non-slip, softer flooring in high-risk floor zones.
高风险地板区域安装防滑软地板。

Use patients' ideas: day-room activity – 'talk about falls over tea'.
利用患者的想法：日间活动——"茶余饭后谈论跌倒"。

Use families' expertise: e.g. grandchildren to assess risk and 'keep grandma/grandpa safe'.
利用家人的专业知识：例如让孙子、孙女评估风险，"保护奶奶、爷爷的安全"。

Patient or family 'falls champions'.
记录患者或家属为"跌倒冠军"。

Reduction in admissions and length of stay: fewer patient days, fewer falls.
减少住院人数和住院时间：住院天数越少，跌倒次数越少。

From what baseline data tells us
基线数据报告

Review trends: where and when do most falls occur?
趋势回顾：大多数跌倒发生在何时何地？

What do patient, family and staff stories tell us?
患者、家人和员工的故事告诉我们什么？

What do we learn by observation?
通过观察我们学到了什么？

number tested first.

• *Forced rank:* Here, each team member ranks the available options from 1 to last. Once everyone has ranked, totals are tallied with the winning option having the lowest total. This method is most practical with a smaller number of options in play – 8 or fewer.

Various tools and approaches can be also be used to support thinking that is more likely to lead to fundamental, rather than incremental, change. These include:

• Patient (or customer) focus: Going beyond the usual methods of survey, interview and focus group, spending time shadowing or in structured observation of patients; setting unrealistic goals and asking 'what would have to be true' to reach them; visualising the ideal setting.

• Co-design and co-production with patients and families: Here, patients and families are members of the improvement team alongside professionals. Given that nearly all healthcare interactions follow a 'service' rather than a 'product' logic, this has many benefits (Batalden et al., 2016).

• Using change concepts as provocations to promote newthinking: The Improvement Guide lists 72 distinct change concepts including: eliminating waste, improving work-flow, managing variation and avoiding error, better management of cycle times, better customer service, improving supply chain and better product/service design.

A further aspect of developing solutions is to focus on areas with greatest potential impact. Here, Pareto analysis is helpful, ranking attributes from the most commonly occurring to the least. Figure 8.1 shows an example Pareto analysis of falls by type of hospital ward. Improvement work should focus initially on one of the wards in the categories with the highest number of falls. This concept is sometimes called the '80/20 principle' – that 80% of events stem from 20% of the causes, and that 80% of the benefit can bederived by focusing on these. In this example, not surprisingly, the greatest benefit is likely to be accrued through work with Care of the Elderly and Acute Medicine.

有效。然后计票,得票数最多的先测试。

• 强制排名:在此,每个团队成员将可用选项从 1 到最后进行排名。一旦每个人都进行了排名,统计总数,总得分最低的选项获胜。在选项较少（8 个或更少）时,这种方法最为实用。

各种工具和方法也可用于提供更可能导致根本性而非渐进性变革的思维,其中包括:

• 关注患者（或客户）:超越通常的调查、访谈和焦点小组方法,花费时间跟随或对患者进行结构化观察;设定不现实的目标,并问如何才能实现它们;想象理想的环境。

• 与患者和家属共同设计制作:在这里,患者、家属与专业人员都是改进团队的成员。鉴于几乎所有医疗卫生互动都遵循"服务"而非"产品"的逻辑,因此会产生很多收益（Batalden 等,2016 年）。

• 利用变革概念激发新思维:《改进指南》列出了 72 个不同的变革概念,包括消除浪费、改进工作流程、管理变化和避免错误、更好地管理周期、更好的客户服务、改进供应链和更好的产品 / 服务设计。

开发解决方案的另一个方面是将重点放在具有最大潜在影响的领域。在这里,帕累托分析非常有用,可以将属性从最常发生到最少发生进行排名。图 8.1 显示了按医院病房类型对跌倒进行的帕累托分析的示例。改善工作应首先着重于跌倒次数最多的病房。这个概念有时被称为"80/20 原理",即 80% 的事件源于 20% 的原因,而 80% 的收益可以经由这些原因获得。在此示例中,毫不奇怪,老年护理与急症医学的工作会获得最大的收益。

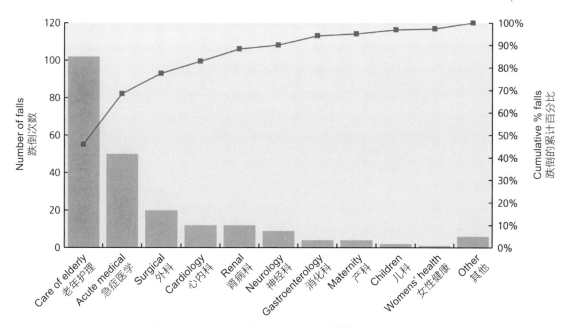

Figure 8.1 Example: Pareto analysis of falls by ward type

图 8.1   示例：按病房类型划分的跌倒的帕累托分析

Testing solutions

Once the team has prioritised what it wants to test, it now needs to test it effectively and efficiently. The best known, most widely adopted and most extensively researched testing model in healthcare is the 'PDSA' or Plan Do Study Act cycle, part of the Model for Improvement (Langley et al., 2009), stemming from the question 'What change can we make that will result in improvement?' Although this section will focus on the PDSA cycle, various other models are available all of which share the same basic approach of iterative testing, learning, refinement and retesting. See Chapter 4.

An advantage of the PDSA cycle is that many clinicians find it intuitive and simple to understand at a conceptual level. Figure 8.2 adds detail on what should be considered in each of the cycle's four phases. Some experience of using the method, discipline and effort are required to use the PDSA cycle effectively.

The seeming simplicity of the cycle itself can actually create challenges: often what happens is simplistic application of a sophisticated and powerful approach. Typical issues with how PDSA is applied in healthcare settings include (Reed and Card, 2016):

测试解决方案

一旦团队确定了要测试内容的优先级，现在就需要有效地测试它。在医疗保健领域，最著名、采用和研究最广泛的测试模式是 PDSA，即"计划 – 执行 – 研究 – 行动"循环，这是改进模型的一部分（Langley 等，2009 年），源于"什么样的变革才能导致改进？"这一问题。尽管本节将重点讨论 PDSA 循环，各种其他模式也都可用，所有这些模式采用相同的迭代测试、学习、细化和重新测试的基本方法。参见第 4 章。

PDSA 循环的一个优点是，许多临床医生发现它在概念层面上直观且易于理解。图 8.2 增加了 4 个循环阶段中每个阶段应考虑的细节。要有效使用 PDSA 循环，需要了解使用方法、规程并有工作经验。

循环本身看似简单，但实际上可能带来挑战：通常情况下，所发生的是复杂而强大方法的简单应用。PDSA 如何应用于医疗环境，其典型问题包括（Reed 和 Card，2016 年）：

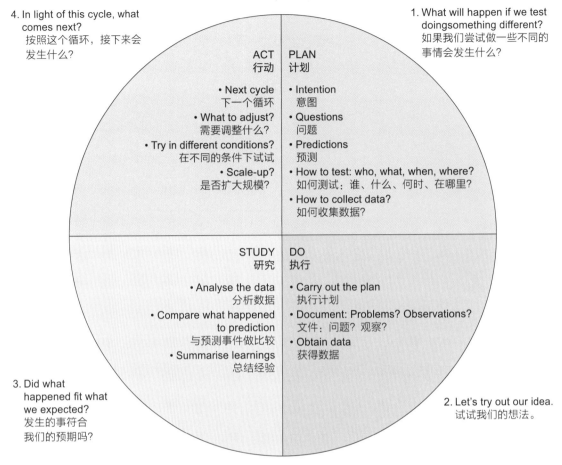

4. In light of this cycle, what comes next?
按照这个循环，接下来会发生什么？

1. What will happen if we test doingsomething different?
如果我们尝试做一些不同的事情会发生什么？

ACT 行动
- Next cycle 下一个循环
- What to adjust? 需要调整什么？
- Try in different conditions? 在不同的条件下试试
- Scale-up? 是否扩大规模？

PLAN 计划
- Intention 意图
- Questions 问题
- Predictions 预测
- How to test: who, what, when, where? 如何测试：谁、什么、何时、在哪里？
- How to collect data? 如何收集数据？

STUDY 研究
- Analyse the data 分析数据
- Compare what happened to prediction 与预测事件做比较
- Summarise learnings 总结经验

DO 执行
- Carry out the plan 执行计划
- Document: Problems? Observations? 文件：问题？观察？
- Obtain data 获得数据

3. Did what happened fit what we expected?
发生的事符合我们的预期吗？

2. Let's try out our idea.
试试我们的想法。

Figure 8.2 Using the PDSA cycle for discovering changes that work. Source: Adapted from Langley et al. (2009)
图 8.2 使用 PDSA 循环发现有效的变革。资料来源：调整自兰利等（2009 年）

- Focus only (or predominantly) on the PDSA cycle itselfwithout adequate preparation – for example, in issue identification, process/system analysis or test development – or, more broadly, failure at an organisational level to invest in supports which enable teams to deploy the cycle to best effect – ranging from improvement training to access to improvement expertise.
- Insufficient focus on the 'Plan' element: running a seriesof rapid PDSA cycles doesn't mean jumping in without preparation or planning. The action-focus and fast-pace of healthcare delivery (and frequent conviction that 'we know what the answers are') can lead to rushing in with- out adequate preparation – the reverse of the 'planning paralysis' described above. For example, what exactly is the test, what are the

- 在没有充分准备的情况下，仅（或主|要）关注 PDSA 循环本身，例如，问题识别、过程与系统分析或测试开发，或者更广泛地讲，在组织层面上未能投资支持团队部署，以达到最佳效果——从改进培训到获得改进专业知识。
- 对"计划"的关注不够：运行一系列快速的 PDSA 循环并不意味着没有准备或计划就跳进去。专注于行动和快速的医疗服务（以及经常认为"我们知道答案是什么"）可能会导致没有充分准备就仓促进入，这与前面提到的"计划瘫痪"刚好相反。例如，测试到底是什么，测试的条件是什么，测试中谁会做什么，什么时候做，如何测量

conditions, who will do what and when in the test, and how will we measure and document findings?

- Insufficient focus on the 'Study' element: The iterative refinement of theory is core to the PDSA approach, yet often overlooked in practice, leading to overgeneralisation and premature scale-up.

In a systematic literature review of application of the PDSA cycle, Taylor et al. (2014) found that in over 400 published studies using PDSA cycles, only 18% met inclusion criteria for deploying all key features of the method, including prediction-based testing of stated theory, test documentation and recording data overtime and initial small-scale testing. Of these 18%, only 19% fully documented the application of a series of iterative cycles.

Building knowledge through linking sequential PDSA cycles

Central to the PDSA approach is linking together a series of changes in a 'learning ramp' (see Figure 8.3). Initially very small-scale tests of theories and ideas of what might drive improvement are run. Subsequent cycles follow, informed by what was discovered in earlier cycles. Knowledge is built sequentially with each cycle and typically, over time, the complexity and scale of tests increases. Changes are tested under a variety of conditions toward discovering solutions which represent improvements that are sustainable in daily practice. For example, in the falls example used in Box 8.1, if staff determined there was an issue with patien slipping and prioritised testing changes focusing on non-slip flooring or socks, this would initially be done 'on one day for one bay'. Then, based on the results, the changes would next be refined and tested under different conditions, such as: in another bay, with different staff, at night or at the weekend rather than during the usual working day, on another ward. Implementation, embedding and sustaining these changes as new usual ways of working follows this discovery phase. They represent a distinct phase of improvement which is the focus of Chapter 10.

Note that Figure 8.3 is an idealised and simplified description of what, in practice, is messier. Real-life scale-up involves false starts, revisions, plateaus and regrouping, rather than

和记录结果。

- 对"研究"的关注不足：理论的迭代完善是 PDSA 方法的核心，但在实践中经常被忽略，导致过度宽泛，过早地扩大规模。

在对 PDSA 循环应用的系统文献回顾中，泰勒等（2014 年）发现，在使用 PDSA 循环的 400 多个已发表研究中，只有 18% 符合该方法所有关键特征的纳入标准，包括基于预测的理论测试，测试文件和记录数据超时和初始小规模测试。在这 18% 中，只有 19% 充分记录了一系列迭代循环的应用。

通过连接顺序 PDSA 循环积累知识

PDSA 方法的核心是将"学习坡度"中的一系列变革链接在一起（图 8.3）。最初进行的是针对可能推动改进的理论和想法做小规模的测试。随后的循环跟随先前循环中发现的信息。知识是在每个循环中顺序建立的，通常随着时间的推移、测试的复杂性和规模会增加。在各种条件下对变革进行测试，以发现在日常实践中可持续改进的解决方案。例如，在框 8.1 中使用的跌倒示例中，如果工作人员确定存在患者滑倒的问题，并将测试重点放在防滑地板或袜子上，则最初应在"一天一个隔间"进行测试。然后，根据结果，接下来将对这些变革进行细化，并在不同的条件下进行测试。例如，在另一个病房，由不同的工作人员在晚上或周末，而不是在工作日进行测试。在探索阶段过后，实施、嵌入和维持这些变革，作为新的常规工作方式。它们代表了一个独特的改进阶段，这是第 10 章的重点。

请注意，图 8.3 是一个理想化的简化描述，实践起来会更为混乱。现实生活中规模的扩大涉及错误的出现、修订、停止和重组，而不是"平稳发展"（Ogrinc 和 Shojania，

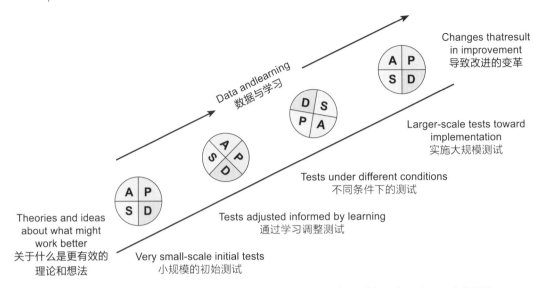

Figure 8.3 Repeated, linked use of PDSA cycles. Source: Adapted from Langley et al. (2009)
图 8.3 PDSA 循环的重复、链接使用。资料来源：参考自兰利等（2009 年）

the smooth progression depicted (Ogrinc and Shojania, 2013).

Sustainability is best approached by ensuring the right people are involved in the work from the start. Bringing together a wide multiprofessional team to drive improvement work, with patients and families, creates a powerful force for sustainability, and organisations are increasingly having senior leaders function as sponsors or advocates for improvement work. Another important angle is ensuring the scope of the work (and measurement approach) include financial/ return on investment elements.

Ethical considerations

A frequent question around improvement work is whether ethics approval is required. This is a complex area, and every organisation should have internal governance arrangements for this. That said, improvement is different from research, centring on how to ensure the best care as defined by current evidence, generated by research, actually reaches every patient, every time. Changes have traditionally been made to care processes and systems in rather haphazard, even unplanned ways and without careful measurement. We can think of improvement as bringing intentionality and transparency to such changes. Combined with the principle of 'start small and build on what works', this should

2013 年）。

最好从一开始就确保让合适的人参与工作，以实现可持续发展。组建一支庞大的多专业团队，与患者和家人一起推动改进工作，为可持续发展累积强大力量，并且组织高级领导者担任改进工作的发起者或倡导者。另一个重要角度是确保工作范围（和测量方法）涵盖财务和投资回报。

伦理考量

改进工作的一个常见问题是，是否符合伦理道德要求。这是一个复杂的领域，每个组织都应该为此制订内部管理安排。也就是说，改进不同于研究，其中在于如何确保研究产生的现有证据所定义的最佳护理能真正惠及所有患者。传统上对护理过程和系统的改变是随意的，甚至是无计划的，没有仔细测量。我们可以把改进看作是给这些变革带来意向性和透明度。结合"从小处做起，以有效为基础"的原则，这应该让患者、专业人员和系统内的领导者确信，道德考量是改

reassure patients, professionals and system leaders that ethical considerations are front and centre in good improvement work. Put another way, it seems unethical not to know how reliable our care processes are, how much variation exists in the care provided and how to harness the best tools and intelligence we have to deliver better care to every patient, every time.

The power of the method and its resonance with clinicians

As we have seen, systematically applying a model by which well-considered solutions are prioritised, tested, refined and then adopted, adapted or abandoned, linked to measurement of what matters to patients and staff, is a powerful and essential element of discovering what works in your context. There are additional benefits to this method, including:

- It is an inherently human, participatory activity. Usedwell, the tools described above can be used to break down hierarchies, give voice to everyone and build effective teams, reinforced by mutual trust.
- It allows teams to run tests which they predict may fail,with a safety net – this may be important in creating alignment or challenging an entrenched point of view.
- It enables teams, in a controlled way, to make changeswith minimal risk of harm to patients or wasted resource.

Finally, for clinicians trained in science, the method is intuitive: 'Plan Do Study Act' is analogous to Francis Bacon's scientific method of 'Hypothesis Test Measure Retest' – the key difference being the speed with which cycles are run. It also matches how clinicians think in approaching the diagnosisand treatment of patients: they don't run a full history and examination on a child with abdominal pain and nausea before starting to form a perspective about the likely diagnoses and the characteristics which will lead to supporting one above another. If the initial pattern supports a diagnosis of appendicitis, history and examination are tuned to testing that as the favoured diagnosis – and based on the findings, appendicitis is adopted, adapted or abandoned as a working diagnosis. Similarly, if a patient has raised blood pressure, a physician will try a series of approaches, from lifestyle and diet to pills, singly or in

进工作良好的首位和中心。换言之，如果不知道我们的护理流程有多可靠，所提供的护理存在多大差异，以及如何利用最好的工具和智慧为每位患者提供更好的护理，这似乎是不道德的。

该方法的强大功能及与临床医生的互动

正如我们所看到的，系统地应用一个模式，通过该模式，经过深思熟虑的解决方案获得优先测试、完善，然后被采纳、调整或放弃，并与对患者和工作人员均重要的事情相联系，这可以发现环境中什么在起作用。这种方法还有其他收益，包括：

- 这是一种人类固有的参与性活动。如果使用得当，上述工具可以用来打破等级制度，让每个人都有发言权，有助于建立有效的团队，并在信任的基础得到巩固。
- 允许团队使用安全的网络运行预测可能会失败的测试，这对于建立趋同的思想或挑战顽固的观点来说很重要。
- 让团队能够以可控的方式做出变革，并将患者受到伤害或资源浪费的风险降至最低。

最后，对于受过科学训练的临床医师来说，这种方法是直观的："计划－执行－研究－行动"类似于弗朗西斯·培根的科学方法"假设－测试－测量－重新测试"，关键区别在于循环运行的速度。这也符合临床医生在患者会诊时的想法：起初形成一些可能的诊断，在获得可以证实的观点之前，没有对腹痛、恶心的儿童进行全面的病史检查和身体检查。如果最初的症状支持阑尾炎这一诊断，则应调整病史检查和身体检查，并测试首选的诊断，根据测试结果，采用、调整或放弃阑尾炎这一诊断。同样，如果患者血压

combination, titrating the treatment to the patient's physiological response. So it is with quality improvement.

高，医生将尝试从生活方式、饮食到药物等一系列方法，单独或组合使用，根据患者的生理反应调整治疗方案。质量改进也是如此。

References
参考文献

Batalden M, Batalden P, Margolis P et al. (2016) Co-production of healthcare services. *BMJ Quality and Safety*, 25, 509-517.
Gawande A. (2008) *Better: A Surgeon's Notes on Performance*, London, Picador.
Langley GJ, Moen RD, Nolan KM et al. (2009) *The Improvement Guide*, 2nd edn, San Francisco, CA, Jossey Bass.
Ogrinc G and Shojania K. (2013) Building knowledge, asking questions. *BMJ Quality and Safety*, 23, 265-267.
Reed JE and Card AJ. (2016) The problem with Plan-DovStudy-Act cycles. *BMJ Quality and Safety*, 25,147-152.
Taylor MJ, McNicholas C, Nicolay C et al. (2014) Systematic review of the application of the plan-do-study-act method to improve quality in healthcare. *BMJ Quality and Safety*, 23, 290-298.

Further reading and resources
深度阅读与相关资源

Institute for Healthcare Improvement Toolkit: How to Improve? Available at: www.ihi.org/resources/Pages/HowtoImprove/ default.aspx (accessed 2 May 2019).
Jones B, Vaux E and Olsson-Brown A. (2019) How to get started in quality improvement. *British Medical Journal* 364, k5408.
Quality Improvement Made Simple: What Everyone Should Know about Health Care Quality Improvement (2013). The Health Foundation Quick Guide. The Health Foundation, London.

第9章 | 测量

Paul Sullivan

Consultant in Acute Medicine, Chelsea and Westminster Hospital, London, UK
Honorary Senior Lecturer in Improvement Science, Imperial College, London, UK

OVERVIEW
概述

- Data, both quantitative and qualitative, is vital for understanding the impact of any change made.
  数据，无论是定量还是定性，对于理解变革的影响都是至关重要的。
- Three main types of measures are used: outcome, process and balancing measures.
  主要使用了3种类型的测量方法：结果测量、过程测量和平衡测量。
- Use just enough sequential, time - series data for the measurement of the impact of any change.
  使用足够的连续时间序列数据来测量变革产生的影响。
- Embed measurement as part of business as usual by using data collected routinely or add data collection to existing processes.
  使用常规收集的数据或将数据收集添加到现有流程中，将测量作为业务的一部分嵌入流程。
- Present collected data in a run chart or statistical process control chart to show variation over time and to determine whether changes made are leading to improvement and the intended goal.
  在运行图或统计过程控制图中显示随时间变化的数据，确定所做的变革是否导致改进，是否达到预期目标。

Introduction

'Without data you're just another person with an opinion.' (W. Edwards Deming)

Data is vital for improvement. Data allows us to rise above anecdote, to describe the current situation scientifically, to understand what needs fixing, and what we should prioritise. More importantly, data tells us when a real improvement has been achieved and, when we do serial tests of change, which ones have worked. There are rare instances where a change is huge and obvious; for example, where significant resource has been added and a waiting list goes from months to days. However, changes are almost always too small to 'see with the naked eye' and data is needed to determine the impact that any change has had. Presenting real-time

引言

"没有数据，你只是一个有意见的人。"（爱德华兹·戴明）

数据对改进至关重要。数据使我们能够越过奇闻轶事，科学地描述当前的情况，了解需要解决的问题，以及应该优先考虑的问题。更重要的是，数据告诉我们什么时候实现了改进，当我们对变革进行一系列测试时，哪些测试有效。很少有变革是巨大而明显的，例如投入了大量资源后，等待列表从几个月变为几天。然而，变革几乎总是太小，无法用肉眼看到，需要数据来确定变革所产生的

data to teams focuses attention, makes deficits clearly visible and motivates action. Showing improvement with data creates momentum and enthusiasm. Often, feeding data back to a team is allthat's needed to drive improvement. Conversely, a project that lacks data will struggle to hold attention.

This chapter focuses on how to use both quantitative and – to a lesser extent – qualitative data to understand if change is leading to an improvement.

What to measure

It's essential to measure the right thing. Good measures will be strongly linked to your aim and a change in these metrics, in response to an intervention, should reflect how the aim is being achieved. Different types of measures are used which, in the main, are either outcome measures (what matters to patients), process measures (how systems and processes work) or balancing measures (trade-offs).

Outcome measures

There are many facets of quality in healthcare, and these have been discussed in Chapter 1. Some of these can be seen as the 'end product' of care or clinical outcome (e.g. death, mobility after joint replacement), some relate to the patient experience (were you anxious? were you in pain?) and others to patient safety (pressure ulcers, falls). These can be measured directly and are called outcome measures.

Process measures

Often, it can be difficult to collect outcome measures. Consider, for example, trying to increase the number of patients with heart failure prescribed a beta blocker to reduce mortality. If we try to measure mortality, we have to wait years to see the benefit, and may never accrue enough patients – tens of thousands of patients are needed in research trials to see these effects. In this instance, it is impossible to obtain outcome data to provide real-time feedback on any changes made to improve practice. Instead, a better measure might be the number of eligible patients who get the right prescription. This called a process measure. Almost all quality improvement (QI) data relies on process measures.

影响。向团队提供实时数据可以集中注意力，使缺陷清晰可见，并激励其行动。用数据显示改进会产生动力和热情。通常，将数据反馈给团队可以全力推动改进。相反，缺乏数据的项目将很难集中目标。

本章重点介绍如何使用定量和定性数据小范围来了解变革是否会导致改进。

测量什么

测量正确的东西是至关重要的。好的测量标准与目标紧密相连，当目标调整时，测量标准应随之改变。测量标准有不同的类型，主要包括结果测量标准（对患者来说什么重要）、流程测量标准（系统和过程如何工作）或平衡测量标准（权衡）。

结果测量

医疗保健的质量有很多方面，第 1 章已经讨论过。其中一些可以被视为护理或临床的"最终结果"（如死亡、关节置换术后活动），一些与患者体验有关（焦虑、疼痛），还有一些与患者的安全有关（压疮、跌倒）。这些都可以直接测量，称为结果测量。

流程测量

通常，收集用于结果测量的数据可能很困难。例如，考虑增加使用 β 受体阻滞剂的心力衰竭患者人数以降低死亡率。如果我们要测量死亡率，就必须等待数年才能看到结果，并且可能永远不会招募到足够多的患者——研究试验需要成千上万的患者才能观察到效果。在这种情况下，不可能获得结果数据，以提供有关改进实践中任何变革的实时反馈。相反，一个更好的测量标准可能是获得正确处方的合格患者的数量，这称为流程测量。几乎所有质量改进数据都依赖流程测量。

Balancing measures

When making any change, attention should be given to how to capture what might be an unwanted consequence of any well-intended change. With the above example, this might be a reduction in the quality of care for patients with myocardial infarction due to redeployment of cardiac nurse time to heart failure patients.

Box 9.1 illustrates these three different types of measures using the example of improving inappropriate catheterisation.

平衡测量

进行变革时，应注意获取这些意图良好的变革可能造成的不良后果。在上述示例中，由于将心脏护理时间重新分配给心力衰竭患者，而导致心肌梗死患者的护理质量下降。

框 9.1 以改善不当导尿为例说明这三种类型的测量。

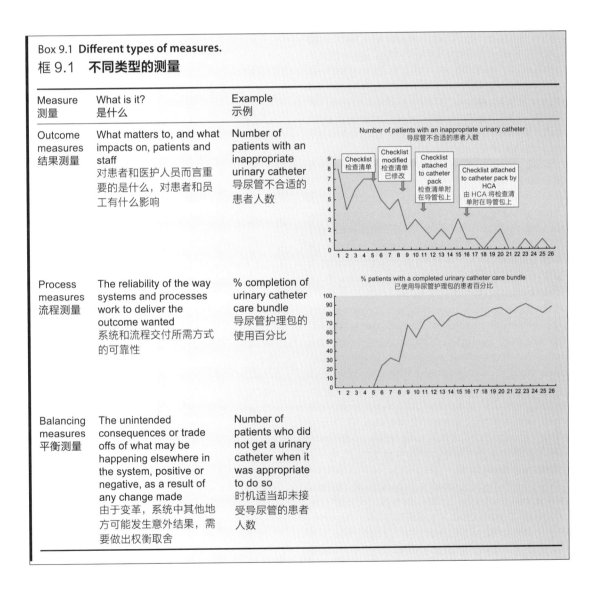

Box 9.1 **Different types of measures.**

框 9.1　**不同类型的测量**

Measure 测量	What is it? 是什么	Example 示例	
Outcome measures 结果测量	What matters to, and what impacts on, patients and staff 对患者和医护人员而言重要的是什么，对患者和员工有什么影响	Number of patients with an inappropriate urinary catheter 导尿管不合适的患者人数	Number of patients with an inappropriate urinary catheter 导尿管不合适的患者人数
Process measures 流程测量	The reliability of the way systems and processes work to deliver the outcome wanted 系统和流程交付所需方式的可靠性	% completion of urinary catheter care bundle 导尿管护理包的使用百分比	% patients with a completed urinary catheter care bundle 已使用导尿管护理包的患者百分比
Balancing measures 平衡测量	The unintended consequences or trade offs of what may be happening elsewhere in the system, positive or negative, as a result of any change made 由于变革，系统中其他地方可能发生意外结果，需要做出权衡取舍	Number of patients who did not get a urinary catheter when it was appropriate to do so 时机适当却未接受导尿管的患者人数	

Getting the right data

A major challenge in QI is getting the right data, and to keep on getting data right through the project and, sustainably, beyond. Whatever is measured needs to reflect the desired achievement. For example, in addressing unacceptably longwaits that seriously impair patient experience, recording average wait time might not be the right measure of success. It might be better to measure the number of patients who wait more than a certain time. If you want to improve communication with patients to improve medication compliance, asking them if they'd recommend you to friends and family would not be the most appropriate measure. If wanting to improve how a certain condition is managed – for example, hospital acquired pneumonia (HAP) – there should be clarity of what constitutes the definition of HAP and what does not, so the right measures are used and understood by everyone.

Data collected may be either quantitative, qualitative or both.

Quantitative data are easier to express in terms of using counts (e.g. number of infections per month), ratios or rates (e.g. infections per 1000 dialysis days), proportions (e.g. percentage of all patients on a ward this month harmed by a fall) or time between events (e.g. time between never events).

Qualitative data that can be used to understand whether change is leading to an improvement may include collating scale measure data (a numerical rating for outcomes for the individual), coding (compiling the data into sections or groups of information known as themes or codes) as well as narrative information about outcomes. Examples include feedback about experience of care, observation of patients waiting for dialysis transport and patient reported experience measures.

Careful thought should be given to the group of patients included in the data collection. By choosing a group that's much broader than the target group, improvement could be diluted and hidden, and time wasted collecting too much data. By choosing a group that doesn't include all the types of patients you want to help, some subgroups might be failing to benefit from your work without your knowing and/ or unintended bias may be introduced into the results.

获得正确的数据

QI 的一个主要挑战是获取正确的数据，且在项目中持续正确地获取数据。无论测量什么，都需要反映预期的成果。例如，在处理严重影响患者体验的事件时，对于难以忍受的长时间等待，记录平均等待时间不是衡量改进的正确标准，而是最好测量等待超过一定时间的患者数量。如果你想改进与患者的沟通以提高服药依从性，询问他们是否会把你推荐给朋友和家人并不是最合适的测量方法。如果想改进某种疾病的管理方式，如医院获得性肺炎（HAP），应该明确什么是 HAP，什么不是，这样每个人都可以理解和使用正确的测量方法。

收集的数据可以是定量的，也可以是定性的，或者两者兼有。

定量数据更容易用计数（如每月感染人数）、比率或比数（如每 1000 个透析天数出现的感染人数）、比例（如本月病房中所有患者因跌倒而受伤的百分比）或事件间隔时间（如从不发生事件的间隔时间）来表示。

可用于了解变革是否导致改进的定性数据包括：量表（对个体结果的数字评级）、编码（将数据汇编成主题或代码的信息节或组）以及结果的叙述性信息。示例包括护理经验的反馈、等待透析转运患者的观察和患者报告的体验。

应仔细考虑纳入数据收集的患者群体。通过选择一个比目标群体更广泛的群体，改进可能会被稀释和隐藏，而且收集太多的数据会浪费时间。如果不小心遗漏了某些患者群体，某些子群体可能无法从你的工作中获益，结果可能会出现意想不到的偏差。

How to measure

The guiding principle here is to use just enough sequential time-series data for real-time measurement of the impact of any change. To ensure sustainability of data collection, measurement should ideally be embedded within 'business as usual' processes either by using data routinely collected, or through adding new data collection processes to one that is already in place. It is important to get this right. Some data may be being collected already for other purposes. This provides an opportunity, and in this situation, data can be retrieved with some confidence from notes or IT systems. Some data requires additional work to record or log it. This is a risk. Most data collection falls down either because people don't record it in the first place, it takes too long to manually trawl through records or promises from an IT department for additional data functionality just don't come through in time.

How to analyse and present findings

Using continuous data – a series of data points over time plotted in order – brings out the story in the data. It allows a change to be detected as it happens. It's much more informative and useful than 'before and after' data. Sometimes a change happens, as a result of a planned intervention you have done, that is so large that no one could miss it on a simple chart. Most often, change may be more subtle and using a run chart or statistical process control chart helps show if variation in an outcome or process over time is random or non-random and whether any changes made are leading to improvement and the intended goal. For these reasons, measurement for QI is different to measurement for research (Box 9.2). The main measurement tools used in QI are the run chart and the Shewhart or statistical process control (SPC) chart (see below).

如何测量

这里的指导原则是使用足够多的连续时间序列数据来实时测量任何变革的影响。为确保数据收集的可持续性，理想情况下，测量应嵌入到已往的流程中，方法是使用常规方法收集的数据，或通过向已有的数据收集流程添加新的数据收集流程。正确处理这一点很重要。一些数据可能已经用于其他目的，这提供了一个机会，在这种情况下，方便从笔记或 IT 系统中检索数据。有些数据需要额外的工作来获取，这是一种风险。如果大多数数据收集都失败了，要么是因为人们没有在第一时间记录下来，要么是因为需要花费太长的时间来手动搜索记录，要么是因为 IT 部门对附加数据功能的承诺没有及时兑现。

如何分析并呈现测试结果

使用连续的按时间顺序绘制的一系列数据点揭示数据中的故事，它允许在发生变化时检测到变化，跟之前和之后的数据相比能提供更多信息，更有用。有时，对于有大的变化没有人会在简单的图表上遗漏。大多数情况下，变化可能更微妙，使用运行图或统计过程控制图有助于显示结果或过程随时间的变化是随机的还是非随机的，以及发生的变化是否会导致改进和实现预期目标。由于这些原因，质量改进测量不同于研究测量（框 9.2）。质量改进中使用的主要测量工具是运行图和休哈特或统计过程控制图（SPC）（参见下文）。

Box 9.2 **Measurement for research vs measurement for improvement.**
框 9.2 **为研究而进行的测量与为改进而进行的测量**

	Measurement for research 为研究而进行的测量	Measurement for improvement 为改进而进行的测量
Purpose 目的	To test a hypothesis and discover new knowledge 检验假设并发现新知识	To bring new knowledge into daily practice 将新知识应用于日常实践
Test 测试	One large test, blinded or controlled 一个大型测试，盲测或受控测试	Many sequential, observable tests 许多连续的、可观察的测试
Biases 偏差	Control for as many biases as possible 尽可能减少偏差	Accept consistent bias from test to test 接受一定范围内的偏差
Data 数据	Sample size calculated for enough statistical power to detect a treatment effect 计算样本量以获得足够的统计数据，以便检测治疗效果	Just enough time-ordered data to learn and inform another cycle of change 按时间排序的数据仅够支持学习并提示另一个变革循环
Duration 持续时间	Can take long periods of time to obtain results; rigid protocol used throughout 可能需要很长时间才能获得结果；始终使用制定严格的协议	Small testing cycles of change; adaptive, iterative design 针对变革的短周期测试；自适应迭代设计
Measurement tool 测量工具	Wide range of statistical tests 广泛的统计测试	Run chart or Shewart control chart 运行图或休哈特控制图

Understanding variation

Common cause variation

To understand how we can detect improvement on a chart, we have to understand variation. Everything shows a degree of variation with time; this is just random, background fluctuation. On Monday, the average waiting time in a clinic might be 25 minutes, on Tuesday, 36 minutes, Wednesday, 22 minutes, and so on. What determines the waiting time? It's the sum of lots of small waits – wait to register, get weighed, get notes ready, wait for the doctor to finish writing up the previous appointment. Each one of these in itself varies – different queue lengths, for example. Adding up all these small, ever present, delays gives the overall wait, and the sum will always vary from patient to patient and from day to day. We call this background fluctuation 'common cause variation'. If nothing in the local system changes – same staffing, same number of patients, same number of doctors, etc., the variation will continue in a similar way – you can predict the wait time will almost always be between this time and that.

理解变异

常见原因变异

为了理解如何在图表上检测改进，我们必须理解变异。一切都随着时间显示出一定程度的变异，这只是随机的背景波动。星期一，诊所的平均等待时间可能是 25 分钟，星期二，36 分钟，星期三，22 分钟，以此类推。什么决定了等待时间？这是许多短暂的等待时间的总和——等待挂号、评估、准备笔记、等待医生完成之前的预约，等等。其中每一个过程本身都有变异，如不同的排队长度。把所有这些短暂的、经常出现的延误加起来，就得到了总的等待时间，而且总的等待时间会因每天的变化而有所不同。我们称这种背景波动为"常见原因变异"。如果自身系统没有任何变化——相同的人员配置、相同的患者数量、相同的医生数量等等，这种变异将以类似的方式继续下去——你预测的等待时间几乎总是在某段时间之内。

Special cause variation

Now think about making a change to the process that really alters the average waiting time. Maybe you dispense with routinely weighing the patients, and this cuts out 10 minutes on average. Now the system is different. When you made the change, there was a data shift that was not part of the usual common cause variation. This is special cause variation.

Which measurement tool to use?

Run chart

The run chart (see Box 9.3) is a graphical display of data in time order based around a median line and uses probability-based rules to help identify whether the variation seen is common cause or special cause. Data points in a stable run in a period let you place the median line, and this helps you detect real changes during your improvement work. Time-ordered charts are a very good way to understand your data as you are getting started. Putting flags or annotations where you made changes gives a clear account of what's working and what didn't work. However, run charts do not display statistical control limits, and are less likely to detect a real change in the data more likely to give false alarms, showing a change and when none has occurred, than SPC charts. When the improvements are reasonably large, a run chart works much the same as SPC. If there is a small improvement, SPC charts are more sensitive than run charts.

An example of an annotated run chart is provided in Figure 9.1. This example shows the number of patients who receive all of five heart failure (HF) bundle elements each week. The median value is used. The improvement after echocardiogram prioritisation is manifested as 7 points in a row above the midline (median). And after the nurse starts visiting the acute medical unit (AMU) there is a dramatic jump in performance. In isolation, such events are sometimescalled 'astronomical data points' and trigger a judgement call about whether they represent an improvement, random variation or something else.

特殊原因变异

现在考虑对流程进行变革，以真正改变平均等待时间。也许你不必对患者进行常规测量，这样平均可以减少 10 分钟。现在系统不同了，当你做出改变时，有一个数据出现偏移，它不属于的常见原因变异，这就是特殊原因变异。

使用什么测量工具

运行图

运行图（见框 9.3 ）是基于中经时间顺序的显示数据图形，并使用基于概率的规则来帮助识别所见变异是常见原因还是特殊原因。一段时间内稳定运行的数据点算出，这有助于改进工作期间检测实际的变化。时间顺序图表是了解数据很好的方式。在进行变革的地方设置标志或注释可以清楚地说明哪些有效，哪些无效。但是，与统计过程控制图相比，运行图不显示统计控制限，不太可能检测到数据中的真实变化，更有可能发出错误警报，在没有发生变化的情况下显示有变化。当改进相当大时，运行图的工作方式与统计过程控制图大致相同。如果改进小，统计过程控制图比运行图更敏感。

图 9.1 提供了带注释的运行图示例。这个例子显示每周接受 5 种心力衰竭束支传导阻滞患者的数量。使用中经数，超声心动图改进后的表现为中线上的 7 个点（中位数）。当护士访问急性医疗单元（AMU）后，其表现有了戏剧性的飞跃。作为一个孤立事件，这种事有时被称为"天文数据点"，并触发判断它们是否代表改进、随机变异或其他事件。

Box 9.3 **Run chart rules for interpretation**

框 9.3   **运行图解释规则**

Rule 1 规则 1 A shift 偏移	A shift on a run chart is six or more consecutive points either all above or all below the median 运行图上的偏移是指至少连续 6 个点全部高于或低于中间值	
Rule 2 规则 2 A trend 趋势	A trend on a run chart is five or more consecutive points all going up or all going down 运行图上的趋势是指至少连续 5 个点全部上升或下降	
Rule 3 规则 3 Runs of unusual patterns 异常模式行差	A run is a series of points crosses the median too many times or too few times (there are tables available that outline the 'normal range') 行差是指一系列点中位数两侧过于分散（有表格列出了"正常范围"）	
Rule 4 规则 4 Astronomical point 天文点	Data points that are obviously, or even blatantly different from all or most of the other values 与所有或大部分值明显不同的数据点	

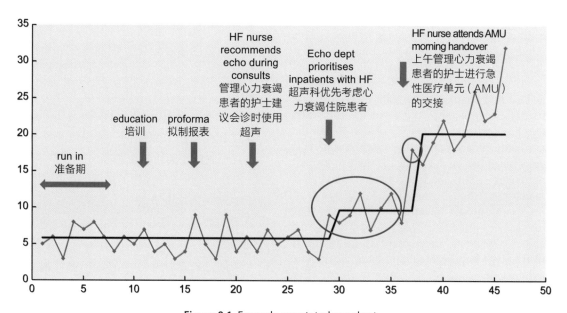

Figure 9.1 Example annotated run chart

图 9.1   注释运行图示例

Statistical process control (SPC) chart

The Shewhart or statistical process control (SPC) chart is a more advanced tool than the run chart. The SPC chart also displays data in time order, but with a mean as the centre line instead of a median. There are upper and lower control limits defining the boundaries within which you would predict the data fall virtually all of the time when there is only common cause variation; that is, when nothing special has happened. SPC charts require software. If this is available, always use SPC rather than a run chart.

During common cause variation, 99.73% of all the points fall between the upper and lower control limits, if your data is from a normal distribution. If the data is from a non-normal skewed distribution, this is approximately true, and so the chart still works. The aim of the chart is to detect special cause, or out of the ordinary variation, which ideally is due to your improvement efforts. It detects patterns in the data that only happen rarely by chance. Outlined in Box 9.4 are the rules for interpreting a SPC chart published by Lloyd Provost (Provost and Murray, 2011). There are other rule sets with minor differences, but they all perform similarly.

If any of the rules are triggered, it's very likely there's been a real change in the system. If this is a positive change and it coincides with something you did as part of an improvement project, you can take the credit. Sometimes a special cause appears for no apparent reason. Occasionally these are false alarms, or they may be due to things happening that you don't know about. Sometimes it can be useful to try to work out what the reason is. A common example is that performance drops off as a result of a key person's absence.

If you think there's been a change in the process, with a rule break, it's time to reset the limits. Now you want to know whether further changes make even more improvement. So you set a new average line and new control limits based on the new, better process. The aim is to make still more changes and show further improvement by breaking a rule again, now against the new chart midline and control limits.

统计流程控制图（SPC）

休哈特图或统计过程控制图（SPC）是比运行图更先进的工具。统计过程控制图也按时间顺序显示数据，但以平均值作为中心线，而不是中间值。控制上限和下限定义了边界，当只有常见原因变异时，几乎可以在所有时间预测数据落在该边界内；也就是说，没有什么特别的事情发生。统计过程控制图需要使用软件，如果可用，请始终使用统计过程控制图而不是运行图。

在常见原因变异过程中，如果数据来自正态分布，99.73%的点落在控制上限和控制下限之间。如果数据来自一个非正态偏态分布，这是近似真实的，因此图表仍然有效。图表的目的是检测特殊原因或异常的变异，理想情况下由于努力改进，很少有偶然数据。框9.4概述了劳埃德·普罗弗斯特发布的统计过程控制图解释规则（Provost和Murray，2011年）。其他规则集有一些细微的差别，但性能都很相似。

如果任何一条规则被触发，很可能是系统发生了真正的变化。如果这是一个积极的变化，并且与改进项目有部分吻合，那么你可以归功于此。有时会出现一个特殊的原因，没有明显的原因。有时这些是误报，或者是由于未知的事情发生所导致。尝试找出原因是有用的，一个常见的例子是，由于关键人物的缺席，绩效下降。

如果流程发生了变化，违反了规则，那么是时候重新设定限制了。如果你想知道进一步的变革是否会带来更多的改进。可以根据新的更好的流程设置新的平均线和新的控制限制。我们的目标是通过再次打破规则来做出更多的改变，并显示进一步的改进。下述设置了新的图表中线和控制极限。

Box 9.4 **Rules for interpreting a control chart**
框 9.4 **控制图解释规则**

Rule 1 规则 1 High or low data point 高或低数据点	A data point outside the control limits 超出控制范围的数据点	
Rule 2 规则 2 Outer third 外 1/3	2 out of 3 consecutive points in the outer thirds of the limits, on the same side 同侧的 3 个连续点中的 2 个在极限外 1/3	
Rule 3 规则 3 Outer two thirds 外 2/3	4 out of 5 consecutive points in the outer two thirds, on the same side 同侧的 5 个连续点中的 4 个在极限外 2/3	
Rule 4 规则 4 A shift 偏移	8 or more points in a row all above or all below the mean 连续 8 个及以上点全部高于或低于平均值	
	6 or more points in a row increasing or decreasing 连续 6 个或更多点上升或下降	
Rule 5 规则 5 A trend 趋势	There are also rules that tell you when something odd has happened to the data, other than a shift in the average performance 除了超出平均表现的变化外，还有一些规则可以指出何时数据发生异常情况	
Rule 6 规则 6 Multiple systems 多系统	8 consecutive points with no points in the inner third, nearest the midline. This means it's likely you have two separate systems mixed together 连续 8 个点，最靠近中线的内 1/3 区域没有点。这意味着可能有 2 个独立的系统混合在一起	
Rule 7 规则 7 Variability reduced 可变性降低	15 consecutive points in the inner third – indicating that variability has reduced since baseline 内 1/3 中有 15 个连续点——表明变异性自基线检查以来有所降低	

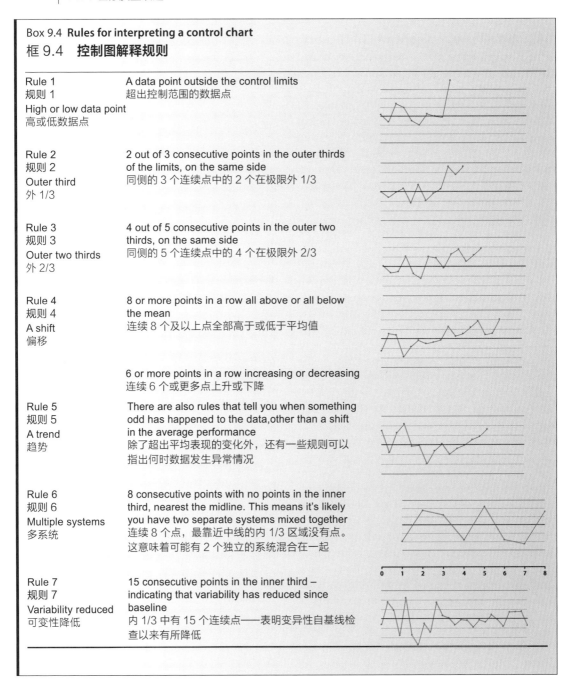

An example of an annotated statistical process control chart is given in Figure 9.2. The same example is used; that is, the chart shows the number of patients who receive all five of the heart failure bundle elements each week. The black line shows the average (mean), red shows the control limits and the pink lines represent one standard deviation (SD). There is an initial run in phase when no changes are being made;

图 9.2 给出了带注释的统计过程控制图示例。使用了与运行图相同的示例，也就是说，图表显示每周接受 5 种心力衰竭束支阻滞治疗的患者人数。黑线表示平均值，红线表示控制限，粉线表示一个标准差。当没有变革发生时，有一个初始磨合阶段，这提供了设置平均线和控制极限的数据。注释显示了干

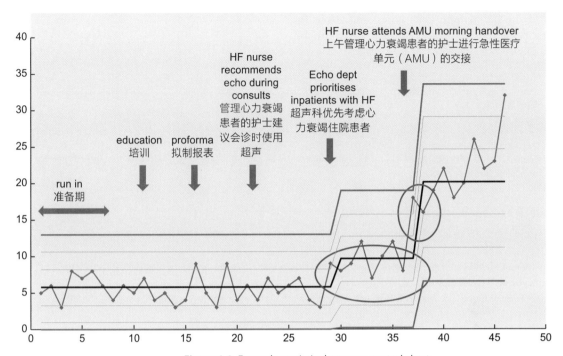

Figure 9.2 Example statistical process control chart

图 9.2　统计流程控制图示例

this provides data to set the average line and the control limits. The annotations show the timing of interventions. Early interventions failed to impact performance, then the reprioritisation of echocardiogram booking resulted in an improvement, evidenced by 8 points in a row above the level of the original average line. Further improvement resulted after the heart failure (HF) nurse started looking for patients on the acute medical unit (two of three points outside the 2SD line).

预的时间。早期干预措施未能达到疗效，新的超声心动图预约规则导致了改进，表现为连续 8 个点高于原来的平均线水平。管理心力衰竭患者的护士在急性医疗单元找到患者后（2SD 线外 3 个点中的 2 个点），情况进一步好转。

Summary

A clear goal and a measurement process are needed to determine if investment in your improvement effort has made a difference. For each measure, consideration should be given to the ease with which data is available and how easy it is to gather. Evidence of outcomes can take a long time. To ensure movement in the right direction, process measures can be very helpful. Imperfect data is better than no data at all and measurement shouldn't stop when you reach your goal. Visibility of continuous measurement in a run or SPC chart will maintain awareness of your improvement endeavour,

总结

需要一个明确的目标和测量过程来确定所推动的改进工作是否产生了效果。对于每项措施，都应考虑数据的易用性和收集的容易程度。证明结果的证据可能需要很长时间才找到。为了确保朝着正确的方向前进，流程措施非常有用。不完美的数据总比没有数据好，当你达到目标时，测量不应该停止。始终利用运行图或统计过程控制图并持续测量将保持努力改进的意识，激励团队继续前进，在快速发现偏差后采取行动。

motivate the team to keep going and allow for any deviations to be picked up and acted upon quickly.

References
参考文献

Provost LP and Murray S. (2011) *The Healthcare Data Guide. Learning for Data for Improvement,* San Francisco, Jossey - Bass.

Further reading and resources
深度阅读与相关资源

Institute of Healthcare Improvement. *Run charts*. Available at: www.ihi.org/resources/Pages/Tools/RunChart.aspx (accessed 8 October 2019).

NHS Improvement. *Statistical Process Control Tool*. Available at: https://improvement.nhs.uk/resources/statistical-process-control-tool/ (accessed 7 October 2019).

NHS Education for Scotland. *Measurement Plan*. Available at: https://learn.nes.nhs.scot/3138/quality-improvement-zone/ qi-tools/measurement-plan (accessed 7 October 2019).

Solberg L, Mosser G and McDonald S. (1997) The three faces of performance measurement: improvement, accountability, and research. *The Joint Commission Journal on Quality Improvement,* 23 (3), 135-147.

Chapter 10

Embedding and Sustaining a Solution

嵌入和维持解决方案

John Dean

Clinical Director for Quality Improvement and Patient Safety, Care Quality Improvement Department, Royal College of Physicians, London, UK

Consultant Physician East Lancashire Hospitals NHS Trust, Blackburn, UK

OVERVIEW
概述

- Up to 70% of quality improvement interventions don't sustain after one year; plan for sustainability from the start.

  高达 70% 的质量改进干预措施在 1 年后无法持续，所以从一开始就要规划其可持续性。

- Focus on the benefit to patients and staff, not just the intervention.

  关注患者和员工的利益，而不仅仅是干预。

- Ensure there is someone to champion the solution.

  确保有人支持解决方案。

- Continue to measure impact and report into normal systems, building the solution into normal workflows.

  持续测量效果并向系统报告，将解决方案构建到正常工作流程中。

- If circumstances change, adapt the solution.

  如果情况发生变化，调整解决方案。

Why improvements don't sustain.

为什么改进不能持续

Between 33% and 70% of quality improvement initiatives are not sustained one year after implementation (Øvretveit, 2003). And this figure may well be higher for improvement projects undertaken by students or health professionals in training. There are many reasons why an intervention isn't sustained; most commonly because the implementation phase is stopped too early, before it is really known whether the intervention has been successful. We need to be sure that a change in a process of care has shown an effect on the outcome of care before we move on from the implementation phase of improvement work. We also need to know that the measure we chose to demonstrate the effect of the intervention has remained stable for a few weeks or months, ideally staying within new control limits, with common cause

33%~70% 的质量改进计划在实施 1 年后无法持续（Øvretveit，2003 年）。对于学生或医疗专业人员在培训中实施的改进项目，这个数字可能更高。改进不能持续的原因有很多，最常见的原因是，在真正知道改进是否成功之前，就在实施阶段过早停止。在改进工作实施阶段开始之前，需要确保护理过程中的变革对护理结果产生了影响。还需要保证用来证明改进效果的措施在数周或数月内保持稳定，理想情况下应保持统计过程控制图上的数据在新的控制范围内，并且存在常见原因变异（参见第 9 章）。

variation, on a statistical process control chart (see Chapter 9).

Sustaining change usually comes down to embedding new patterns of human behaviour, so understanding what influences and motivates those behaviours helps us in planning what to do. People want to do the right thing, theeasiest thing, and the thing that is most likely to have benefit. When implementing and sustaining a change the three components that will influence whether the change, or the benefits, are maintained are the:

- **intervention**
- **people** who need to use the intervention
- **environment** in which the intervention needs to happen.

We can increase the likelihood of sustainability by addressing all three components. Figure 10.1 expresses these diagrammatically in terms of 'process', 'staff' and 'organisation'.

持续的变革通常是一种嵌入人类行为的新模式，因此了解其影响并激励这些行为有助于做规划。人们希望做正确的、最简单的以及最有可能受益的事情。在实施和维持变革时，会影响变革或利益的 3 个组成部分是：

- 干预措施。
- 需要使用干预措施的人。
- 需要实施干预措施的环境。

通过处理所有这 3 个方面的问题，可以提高可持续性。图 10.1 用"过程""人员"和"组织"的形式示意性地表示了这些。

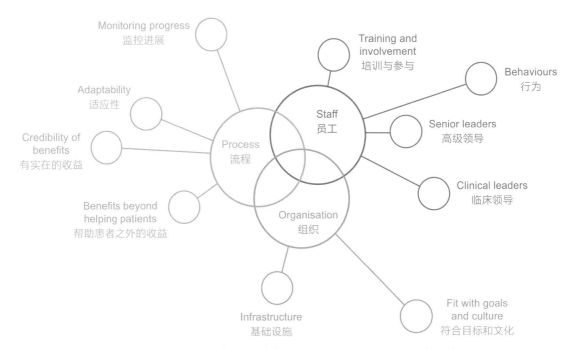

Figure 10.1 A model of sustainability. Source: NHS Improvement (2018)

图 **10.1**　可持续性模式。资料来源：NHS 改进部门（2018 年）

The intervention

The complexity of an intervention will affect how easily it is maintained. The simpler it is, the more likely it is to be sustained in practice. This is often achieved by breaking down an intervention into component parts during the testing phase. How easy a given intervention is to implement can be assessed through successive Plan Do Study Act (PDSA) cycles during which the views of staff and colleagues can be canvassed.

Framing the results of an intervention as benefits that are important to people, particularly to patients and staff, is also key to its sustainability. The benefits of the intervention need to be clear. If they are easily observed in daily practice, that helps. Ideally the intervention makes the best thing to do, the easiest thing to do. It is important to ensure that staff using the intervention, and anyone else involved, are kept informed about the results. This requires planning measurements that make clearly visible the results of every one's endeavours.

If staff need new skills or knowledge to complete the intervention, then training or awareness programmes will need to be arranged and be ongoing. It may be possible to incorporate such trainings into induction.

If the intervention fits naturally into normal workflows, it will become part of a routine and not seen as an add-on extra. A new intervention may also help reduce other daily work and if it is similar to other routine tasks, it is useful to see if they can be combined or connected. It may also be possible to create reminders in normal workflows or allied tasks – but beware of pop up or sticker fatigue!

Changing working environments, such as a change in location or staff, are likely to mean that an intervention may need to be adapted to continue to work in practice. Interventions that can be adapted are more likely to be sustained. In doing so we need to consider what the key components of the intervention are that produce the results and be clear that these are preserved in any future adaptation.

The people who use the intervention

Understanding those who will use the intervention and what will make them want to use it is important. There are several types of people

干预措施

干预措施的复杂性将影响其维护的容易程度。干预措施越简单，就越有可能在实践中持续下去。这通常是通过在测试阶段将干预措施分解为多个步骤来实现。通过连续的计划－执行－研究－行动（PDSA）循环，可以评估特定干预措施实施的容易程度，在此期间可以征求职工和同事的意见。

将干预结果归结为对人，尤其是对患者和工作人员而言至关重要的收益，这也是保持其可持续性的关键。干预的效果需要明确，如果在日常实践中容易观察，那就更有帮助。理想情况下，干预是指做最好、最容易的事情。重要的是确保执行干预措施的工作人员以及所有其他参与人员都能随时了解结果。这需要规划测量，以便使每个人努力的结果清晰可见。

如果工作人员需要新的技能或知识来完成干预，则需要安排并持续开展培训或认知宣传。可以将此类培训纳入入职培训。

如果干预措施适合正常的工作流程，它将成为例行工作的一部分，而不是附加措施。一项新的干预措施也可能会减少其他日常工作，如果与其他日常任务相似，则可以查看它们是否可以合并或连在一起。也可以在正常的工作流程或相关任务中创建提醒，但要注意不要提醒次数过多。

变革工作环境，如地点或工作人员的变革，意味着可能需要调整干预措施，以便在实践中继续工作。可以调整的干预措施更有可能持续下去，在这样做的过程中需要考虑干预的哪个关键组成部分产生了效果，这些关键组成部分应在未来的任何调整中都予以保留。

采用干预措施的人

了解哪些人会采用干预措施，以及他们愿意采用干预措施的因素，这一点很重要。

who will use, or benefit from, an intervention. These include those who developed, tested and adapted it during the planned experimentation. They understand the detail and should also know the effects. Commonly they are also day-to-day users. There will also be champions for the intervention, who will continue to make sure it is used, that the benefits are measured and that people know about them. In addition to champions it is also helpful to identify senior people in the organisation who know about the intervention and the impact. They will be able to ask questions about itsreliable use if the outcome of the intervention starts to go off track. Box 10.1 outlines the people who will be involved in the use of the intervention now and in the future, and some key characteristics of each group that need to be borne in mind.

Communication is key to enabling sustainability through engaging the people who will use the intervention. You will notice there is considerable overlap here with how you get people on board with your improvement endeavour as described in Chapter 5. A communication and engagement plan for sustaining the solution needs to be developed, bearing in mind the key audiences in Box 10.1. The communication needs to include:

- What the intervention is and how to use it, including how it should fit into everyday practice.
- The benefits of the intervention and results from the implementation phase, and results from similar work elsewhere.
- How the use and impact will continue to be monitored.
- Who to contact if there are problems.
- Who the champions for the intervention are.

Different formats of communication will be needed for different audiences. For clinical interventions, all members of the multiprofessional team need to be made aware, as they will prompt each other to use them. Incentives and rewards can be similarly nuanced for each group to make sure interventions are used.

It is helpful to identify and agree a process owner both within the team using the intervention, for example on the ward, and if appropriate across the organisation, for example a patient safety or clinical effectiveness lead.

有几种类型的人会采用干预措施，或从中受益，如在实验中制订、测试和调整它的人。他们了解细节，也应该知道效果。通常他们也是日常用户。干预措施也需要有支持者，确保干预措施的实施，衡量其干预效果，并确保人们了解。除了支持者之外，确定组织中有了解并能够影响干预措施者也很有帮助。如果干预的结果偏离轨道，他们能够就干预措施的可靠性提出问题。框 10.1 概述了现在和将来参与使用干预措施的人员，以及需要记住的每个群体的一些关键特征。

为让采用干预措施的人参与进来，沟通是实现可持续改进的关键。您将注意到，这与如何让人们参与改进方面有相当多的重叠，如第 5 章所述。需要制订一项维持沟通和参与计划的解决方案，同时铭记框 10.1 中的关键群体。沟通要点包括：

- 干预措施是什么，如何实施，包括如何在日常实践中应用。
- 干预措施的收益，实施阶段以及其他类似工作的成果。
- 如何持续监控干预措施的推进和影响。
- 出现问题时联系谁。
- 谁是干预措施的支持者。

不同的群体需要不同的沟通方式。对于临床干预，需要让多专业团队的所有成员都了解，因为他们会互相提示使用干预措施。为了确保干预措施的实施，每个小组的激励和奖励措施可能会有类似的细微差别。

在采用干预措施的团队内，例如在病房内，在适当的情况下以及在整个组织内，确定一个流程负责人很有必要，如患者安全或临床有效性负责人。

Box 10.1 **People who use the intervention and important characteristics.**

框 10.1   **采用干预措施的人及其重要特征**

Developers 制订者	Have worked with you as part of your improvement team and been part of the PDSAs. They may have been in your core team, or wider group involved 作为改进团队的一分子与您合作，并成为 PDSA 的一部分。他们可能在您的核心团队中，或者在更外围的团队中参与	• Understand the intervention in detail 详细了解干预措施 • Significant commitment to sustaining 对持续改进做出重要承诺
Champions 支持者	Ideally more than one from each staff group using the intervention and including people who will be working in that place for several years. Include a senior colleague 理想情况下，执行干预措施的每个员工群体中有一人以上是支持者，包括在该场所工作几年的人员，还包括一位资深同事	• Believe strongly in the intervention and its benefit 坚信干预措施及其收益 • Prepared to continue to communicate the benefits 准备好继续宣传这些收益
Messengers 信使	They may be in the clinical area, or outside. They may be your colleagues, who need to know about the intervention, its impact and how to use it, or senior leaders in the organisation who want the impact to be sustained 可能在临床，也可能不在临床。他们可能是您的同事，需要了解干预措施、干预措施带来的影响以及如何使用，或者可能是组织中希望保持这种影响的高级领导	• Know about the intervention and the impact 了解干预措施及其影响 • Good communicators 良好的宣传者 • Trusted and respected by colleagues 同事信任并尊重的人
Followers 跟随者	They will mainly be users but can include people with an interest in the benefit 他们主要是用户，但可以包括对收益感兴趣的人	• Understand the benefits of the intervention, how to use it, and want to use it 了解干预的收益和如何使用，并希望使用它
Other adopters 其他采用者	Need to use the intervention for it to maintain the benefit, and need it to be easy to use in their everyday practice and see it as normal practice 需要使用干预措施来保持收益，并需要在日常实践中易于使用，并将其视为正常做法	• See Figure 10.2 参见图 10.2
Direct users 直接用户	This includes many of the groups above, but in time staff will change, so many of these won't know it's a new intervention, but need to understand how to use it, and the benefits. It needs to be seen as part of their normal practice 这包括上面的许多小组，但随着时间的流逝，员工会有所变化，因此其中许多人不知道这是一项新的干预措施，但需要了解如何使用以及它带来的收益。必须将其视为正常做法	• A wide range of characteristics and behaviours 广泛的特征和行为
Beneficiaries 受益者	Both staff and patients should benefit from the intervention. They need to know that in intervention produces the benefits 工作人员和患者都应从干预措施中受益。他们需要知道干预可以带来的收益	• Will receive and process information in different ways 以各种方式接收和处理信息

The adoption of new practice has been studied and understood for many years. The Rogers diffusion of innovation curve is well known (Rogers, 2011). See Figure 10.2. Recognising which users are in which category can help. Additional emphasis, both on early adopters and 'laggards', will help sustainability.

The environment in which the intervention happens

It is likely that any proposed solution aims to standardise an element of clinical or operational practice. There are characteristics of the environment in which the intervention happens that will make this more or less likely to be sustained. These include:

- the culture of standardisation in practice
- the ways of monitoring quality of care
- whether local leadership embraces quality improvement
- how well organised the environment is
- the consistency of staff within the team and their working practices.

It is important to understand the normal working practices in that particular environment and who does what, so that the intervention can be embedded into those practices. It may be that these practices will need to be adapted to enable your intervention to be done as a matter of routine. It is also essential that the people 'in charge' of the workplace have agreed to use the intervention, that everyone knows who the champions are, there is an agreement over the process owner and they and others can know how to monitor the impact, as outlined above.

采用的新做法已经被研究和理解了很多年。如众所周知的罗杰斯创新扩散曲线（Rogers，2011 年），参见图 10.2。识别用户属于哪个类别会很有用，对早期采用者和"落后者"的突出强调将有助于持续改进。

干预措施实施的环境

提议的任何解决方案可能都旨在使临床或操作实践的要素标准化。干预措施实施的环境特征会或多或少地使这种情况得以持续。包括：

- 实践中的标准化文化。
- 护理质量的监测方法。
- 本地领导是否支持质量改进。
- 环境构建的有多好。
- 团队内员工与其工作相匹配。

重要的是，要了解在特定环境中的正常工作实践由谁来做，这样才能将干预措施嵌入到这些实践中。可能需要对这些实践进行调整，使干预成为例行事务。同样重要的是，工作负责人同意采用干预措施，每个人都知道谁是支持者，与流程负责人达成协议，他们和其他人能够知道如何监控影响，如上面所述的那样。一个关键的成功因素是可视化管理。这意味着，干预措施的实施、应用及其长期的益处对在当地工作的人来说是显而

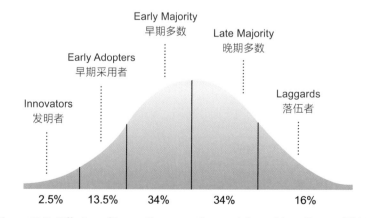

Figure 10.2 Diffusion of innovation curve. Source: Adapted from Rogers (2011)

图 10.2 创新扩散曲线。资料来源：改编自罗杰斯（2011 年）

A key success factor is 'visual management'. That means that how the intervention, its use and ongoing benefits are visible to people working in that place. Making the intervention and impact visible might include:

- Simple 'how to guides' that people can easily access alongside the intervention.
- Including results and ongoing monitoring data on a 'qualityboard'.
- Incorporation into usual clinical governance and reporting systems.

If the intervention is to be used in multiple places, then each place needs some level of understanding. This will be covered in more detail in Chapter 11 on 'Spread'.

Different environments may mean that the intervention and how it is used and monitored need adaptation. The wider environment may also change; there may be a change in staffing roles or senior staff, other changes to practice might influence the intervention and the evidence base may change. So, it is good practice to agree with champions and process owners ongoing curation and what elements of the intervention are key and potentially not changeable, and which could be adapted if necessary to achieve sustainability.

Designing in sustainability

You will have noted that many of the elements that affect sustainability need to be thought about and planned from a very early stage. Leaving this until after initial testing and implementation is too late. We need to think about the sustainability of the intervention from the start. Key elements to be considered early on in a project are shown in Box 10.2. Dependent on the intervention, we also need to consider whether the following are needed for it to become normalpractice:

- Is a business case required? This may be necessary if there are significant costs or risks.
- Do job plans need to be adjusted and negotiated?
- Do other people in the organisation or outside need to agree the intervention as part of normal practice?
- Does it affect the use of facilities or equipment and howthese are managed?

易见的。将干预措施及其影响可视化包括：

- 人们可以在干预过程中能够轻松访问的简单操作指南。
- 在质量委员会中加入结果和持续的监控数据。
- 纳入常规的临床管理和报告系统。

如果要在多处使用干预措施，则对每个地方都需要有一定程度的理解。这将在第 11 章中更详细地介绍。

不同的环境可能意味着需要对干预措施的实施和监控方式进行调整。更外围的环境也可能改变，人员配备或高级人员可能发生变化，实践的其他变化可能会影响干预措施，并且证据基础可能会发生变化。因此，优良做法是与支持者和流程负责人就进行中的管理工作达成一致，确定干预措施的哪些要素是关键且不可变革的，哪些在必要时可以进行调整以实现可持续性。

可持续性设计

你会注意到，许多影响可持续性的因素需要从初始阶段就需要考虑和规划，把它留到初始测试和实现之后就太晚了。我们需要从一开始就考虑干预措施的可持续性。框 10.2 显示了项目早期需要考虑的关键要素。根据干预措施的不同，我们还需要考虑是否需要以下条件才能使其成为常规：

- 是否需要商业案例？如果存在重大成本或风险，这是必要的。
- 工作计划是否需要调整和协商？
- 组织内部或外部的其他人是否同意把干预措施作为常规实践？
- 是否影响设施或设备的使用和管理？

Box 10.2 **Designing in sustainability**

框 10.2 **可持续性设计**

What's the hook? 什么原因	Consider why this change is important to people. Use this in any communications. 考虑一下为什么该变革对人们来说很重要，在所有沟通中都要谈这个 Clarify the problem and need for change, and the potential benefit 明确问题和变革需求，以及潜在的收益
Who can influence success? 谁能影响成功	Get the right people on board or informed from the start, as part of your team or wider stakeholders 组织团队或更广泛的利益相关者，从一开始就让合适的人参与进来或了解情况
Align the initiative with organisational priorities 使计划与组织优先事项保持一致	Find out the organisation's priorities, and if you can make your project part of a wider programme of change 找出组织的优先事项，把项目嵌入变革计划
Combine data and emotional influence 结合数据和情感的影响	Ensure your measurement strategy has the right data and includes patient and staff stories 确保测量策略能拿到正确的数据，包括患者和员工两方面的情况
Make it as simple as possible 尽可能简单	Break down the problem and intervention into component parts and check in your testing phase that it's easy to use or adapt it to be so 将问题和干预措施分解成不同的部分，并在测试阶段检查是否易于使用或调整
Barriers. What could possibly go wrong? 障碍，可能会出什么问题	Identify the barriers to implementation and sustainability and have a plan to manage or minimise them 确定障碍，并制订计划长期实施和管理或将这些障碍分解
Publicity 公开宣传	Make sure people know what you are doing, and why, how it's going, how they can help or influence and what they need to do for success. Make the evidence base clear 确保人们知道你在做什么、为什么做、进展如何，他们如何帮助或影响你，以及他们需要为成功做些什么。明确证据依据
Linking to social movements 与社会运动相联系	Are there any social movements that are working in this area? If so, use social media to publicise your work linked to wider movements for change 在这个地区有什么社会运动在起作用吗？如果是这样，利用社交媒体来宣传你的工作，并将其与更广泛的变革运动联系起来
Keep focused on benefits 专注于收益	Ensure both measurement and communication are focused on benefits to patients and staff, not just the intervention 确保测量和沟通都侧重于为患者和员工带来收益，而不仅仅是出台干预措施

It is also important to consider how long it will take to be sure the intervention is embedded in practice. For doctors in training, and others in rotational roles, it will almost certainly take longer than the time available before being moved to another post. This highlights the importance of working as part of a team when trying to make change happen. Planning for handover should be thought about early on in the life of the project.

同样重要的是要考虑需要多长时间才能确保干预措施落实到实践中。对于医学生和住院医生来说，多数情况下比转移到另一个职位之前需要的时间更长。这突出了在试图做出变革时团队工作的重要性。应在项目早期考虑移交计划。

Ongoing monitoring, measurement and reporting

To ensure that an intervention and its impact are sustained, monitoring needs to be embedded into the organisation's normal governance and reporting structures. This moves us from quality improvement to quality control (see Chapter 1). Measuring the implementation of the intervention or its impact will need to be as straightforward as possible and integrated into other monitoring and reporting practices; for example, quality dashboards. Where that monitoring is reported also needs to be clear (e.g. a departmental clinical governance meeting) as does who will gather the data and do the reporting.

If there are policies, guidelines or standard operating procedures that are linked to the intervention, these need to be updated to include it, and be signed off by the department and organisation.

It is also good to mitigate and plan an intervention for when the measures start to show it is going off track. This is very common, and almost to be expected. Often a short term refocus, with more detailed measurement, and re-raising awareness through good communication is required. The refocus will help to understand where and why using the intervention has slipped, and whether any adaptation is needed.

Changing people's daily working practice is difficult, and ensuring a change is sustained requires determination, planning and resilience. But with a little planning, it can be done and following the steps outlined above will make it more likely that our improvement efforts will reap the desired longer term benefits to patient care and health outcomes (Box 10.3).

Summary

Designing in sustainability right from the start is critical to ensure any improvement endeavour becomes embedded into usual practice. The complexity of any intervention, attention to the context and environment into which change is introduced, the ease with which to measure change and how staff and patients are involved will all determine long-term success.

持续的监控、测量和报告

为了确保干预措施及其影响持续下去，需要将监控纳入组织的正常治理和报告。这使我们从质量改进转向质量控制（见第 1 章）。测量干预措施的执行情况或其影响需要尽可能直接，并纳入其他监控和报告之中、如质量指示板。报告监控的地方也需要明确（例如，部门临床治理会议），以及谁收集数据并进行报告。

如果存在与干预措施相关的政策、指南或标准操作程序，则需要对其进行更新，包括干预措施，并由相关部门和组织签署。

当测量偏离正轨时，缓行并计划干预措施也很有效。这非常普遍，几乎在意料之中。通常需要进行短期的重新评估，进行更详细的测量，并通过良好的沟通重新提高改进意识。重新评估将有助于理解为什么干预措施的实施导致了质量下滑，哪里出现了问题，以及是否需要调整。

改变人们日常的工作习惯是困难的，而要确保一个变革持续下去，就需要决心、计划和应变能力。但只要稍加规划，就可以做到这一点，遵循上述步骤，改进工作更有可能为患者的护理和健康带来预期的长期效益（框 10.3）。

总结

从一开始就进行可持续性设计，对于确保任何改进工作融入常规之中至关重要。干预措施的复杂性、对引入变革的背景和环境的关注、测量变革的容易程度以及员工和患者如何参与都将决定是否可以持续改进。

Box 10.3 Example: improving ward round documentation
框 10.3　示例：改进查房文档

The problem: Geoff and Sue were Foundation Doctors. They were frustrated that when on call and seeing patients on other wards than their own, they couldn't work out what was going on in the care because the documentation of ward rounds, decisions and actions was so variable.

问题：杰夫和苏是基金会的医生。他们感到沮丧的是，值班时如果在自己病房以外的其他病房看病，他们无法了解护理过程中发生了什么，因为查房、决策和治疗的文档非常多变。

Discovery: They had seen a poster at a conference where a ward round proforma had been introduced by junior doctors, and it looked really good. They discovered that the Royal College of Physicians and Royal College of Nursing Ward Rounds Guidance recommended both check lists and structured recording. The example from the conference incorporated both.

发现：他们在一次会议上看到了一张海报，在那里，住院医生介绍了一份查房表，看上去非常不错。他们发现，皇家内科医学院和皇家护理学院查房指南推荐使用检查表和结构化记录，这次的会议将两者结合了起来。

Testing and implementation: They formed a small improvement team of junior doctors, ward nurses, a pharmacist, a physiotherapist and a ward clerk. Each team member asked colleagues what they thought should be on a ward round proforma, and they adapted the one from the conference to test. The consultant on Sue's ward agreed to test it with his team. They scanned the literature for key checks that should happen, and found a number that they made sure were on the form. The form was tested and adapted in Sue's ward. It needed quite a lot of simplification, and clarification on when to use it and where to file it, and where other notes were written. The check lists, diagnosis and actions were the most important parts. The weekend on-call teams and other team members were asked whether it improved their patient assessments, and how frequently the form was being used. A few cases came to light where diagnoses had been missed because of unclear records on other wards. They used these cases to make the case for change. Once working on Sue's ward, then the ward next door wanted to use it. Over the next six months half of the medical wards took up using the proforma following instructions from the Chief of Medicine.

测试和实施：他们成立了一个由住院医师、病房护士、药剂师、理疗师和病房管理员组成的小型改进团队。每个团队成员都表达他们理解的查房表应该是什么，然后他们调整了会议中的查房表来做测试。苏的病房会诊医生同意在他的团队测试。他们浏览了文献资料以查找应进行的关键检查，并找到一个他们确定在表格上的号码。这个表格在苏的病房里进行了测试和修改做了大量简化，并说明何时使用它，在何处归档，以及其他注释是在何处编写的。检查表、诊断和治疗是最重要的部分。周末值班的团队和其他团队成员被问及是否改善了患者评估，以及使用表格的频率。少数病例因其他病房记录不清而漏诊。他们用这些病例来说明做出变革的理由。一开始仅在苏的病房里使用，然后隔壁的病房也想用。在接下来的 6 个月里，一半的病房按照内科主任的指示开始使用这个表格。

Sustainability and monitoring: The final version of the form was agreed by the medical records committee and put on standard ordering for the ward clerks. The ward clerks were given information on ordering, and where to keep the form on the notes trolley. A guide for consultants, nurses, junior doctors and other team members was produced. The patient safety team agreed to monitor the antibiotic review and venous thromboembolism assessment as part of the ongoing audits from the proforma, and these were on the ward quality dashboard. The coding clerks loved the forms and agreed to include this in their part of the junior doctor induction. Sue's consultant agreed to continue to promote the forms use as a champion. This process is now successfully embedded as a business as usual practice.

可持续性和监控：最终版本的表格得到了医疗记录委员会的同意，并为病房管理员提供了订购标准。病房管理员得到关于订购的信息，并将表格放在手推车上的位置。为会诊医生、护士、住院医生和其他团队成员编制了一份指南。患者安全小组同意监测复查抗生素和评估静脉血栓栓塞，作为表格持续审计的一部分，这些都显示在病房质量指示板上。编码员喜欢这些表格，并希望将其纳入住院医生入职培训中。苏的会诊医生同意继续作为支持者推广使用表格。这一流程现在已经成功嵌入到常规业务之中。

References
参考文献

NHS Improvement (2018) Sustainability Model. Available at: https://improvement.nhs.uk/resources/ Sustainability-model-and-guide/ (accessed 19 March 2019).

Øvretveit J. (2003) Making temporary quality improvement continuous: a review of research relevant to the sustainability of quality improvement in health care. *Quality and Safety in Health Care,* 12, 47-52.

Rogers EM. (2011) *Diffusion of Innovations,* 5th edn, London, Simon and Schuster.

Further reading and resources
深度阅读与相关资源

Greenhalgh T. (2018) *How to Implement Evidence-based Healthcare,* Oxford, Wiley.

Kanemahn D. (2011) *Thinking Fast and Slow,* London, Penguin.

Scoville R, Little K, Rakover J, et al. (2016) Sustaining Improvement. IHI White Paper. Cambridge, MA, Institute for Healthcare Improvement. Available at: www.birthtools. org/birthtools/files/ccLibraryFiles/ Filename/000000000310/ IHI-SustainingImprovementWhitePaper.pdf (accessed 19 March 2019).

Aidan Fowler

National Director of Patient Safety, NHS England and Improvement, London, UK

OVER VIEW
概述

- Too much improvement work is undertaken in isolation.
  太多的改进工作是孤立进行的。
- Dissemination and spread are difficult and require planning.
  扩散和传播很困难，需要规划。
- A tendency to distrust interventions 'not invented here' must be actively managed.
  必须积极干预"不是在这里发明的"不信任趋势。
- Communications are a fundamental part of a spread strategy.
  沟通是传播战略的基本组成部分。
- There are many new ways to share knowledge, but traditional conferences and publications still have a role to play.
  分享知识有许多新方法，但传统的会议和出版物仍然可以发挥作用。

Spread and why it may not occur

There is a risk that programmes of quality improvement don't progress beyond individual projects and so the wider benefits for patients and populations are not realised. This is usually played out in two common scenarios: an organisation decides an improvement approach could be of benefit, it builds some capacity and capability (usually too little) and starts to do some improvement work. Alternatively, an enthusiastic individual or small group starts improvement work alone and without support. This is fine as far as it goes and work on a single pathway may well succeed because it is the 'baby' of the project lead, but it doesn't get taken anywhere else; like real babies, we all think ours is beautiful, but it may not have the same appeal to others.

To have greater impact we need to spread ideas; to other units, to other organisations and further afield. 'Too much improvement work is

为什么传播不全会发生

有一种风险是，质量改进计划只局限于单个项目，因此无法让患者和更广泛人群获益。这通常常见于2种情况：一个组织采用的改进方法是有益的，它培养了一些有能力的人（通常太少），并开始做一些改进工作；或者，一个热心的人或小组在没有支持的情况下独自开始改进工作，并且独立进行的工作很可能会成功，因为它是项目负责人的"宝贝"，但在其他任何地方都不会被采用。好比我们都认为自己的孩子很漂亮，但对他人的吸引力可能不一样。

为了产生更大的影响，我们需要把思想传播到其他单位、组织和更远的地方。"在地方层面，孤立地进行了太多的改进工作，

undertaken in isolation at a local level, failing to pool resources and develop collectivesolutions, and introducing new hazards in the process' (Dixon-Woods and Martin, 2016). Spread and scale-up are seldom easy to achieve. The main reason is probably a combination of oversimplification, lift and drop approaches and a tendency to prioritise model fidelity and technical aspects over social or human elements. We also have a tendency to learn from what went well in one place without understanding what failed on the way. Learning from failure is key to planning for success.

Problems of diffusion are not unique to quality improvement, and spread in general – of research, of innovation – can be glacially slow. In healthcare, estimates of lag tend to cluster around a 17-year period of delay (Morris et al., 2011).

Reasons for slow adoption

People take up innovations at a variable rate, and spread starts to take off at about the point where 10% of the population involved have adopted the approach. The 'not invented here' problem means people don't always like adopting others' ideas or believe they will not work. And sometimes people are just too busy with their heads down to see solutions around them. Three other factors are significant: access to knowledge – the ability to find out about something in the first place; readiness of the environment – sometimes referred to as 'soil fertility' which is whether the necessary structures and support are in place for the innovation to work and sustain, and availability of resource – including people, money, methodology knowledge and skills.

Accelerating spread and adoption

What can be done to promote more rapid spread and adoption? Let's take two examples from history: antisepsis and anaesthesia. The global spread of the former took about 30 years, 17 for the latter. Had informed patients had a choice they would, of course, have chosen to have both. So why the difference? One element was particularly influential – and there are many more, including access to the technique, orientation to evidence etc. – and this was the 'what's in it for me?' factor. Anaesthesia meant

无法集中资源并制订集体解决方案，并在此过程中引入了新的危害"（Dixon-Woods 和 Martin，2016 年）。推广和扩散不容易实现，主要原因可能是过于简单化、升降式方法以及倾向于精准模式和技术优先于社会或人为因素。我们也有一种倾向，就是从一个成功的地方学习，而不了解失败的原因。从失败中学习是改进计划成功的关键。

传播问题不是质量改进所独有的，而且从总体上讲，无论是研究还是创新，传播速度都可能很慢。在医疗保健领域，往往滞后 17 年左右（Morris 等，2011 年）。

接受缓慢的原因

人们接受新事物的速度不是一成不变的，大约 10% 的相关人群采用这种方法的时候，新事物的传播就开始了。"不是在这里发明的"意味着人们并不总是喜欢采纳别人的想法，或者认为他们不会成功。有时人们只是埋头工作，看不到周围的解决方案。另外 3 个因素也很重要：获得知识的途径——首先有发现新事物的能力；良好的环境——有时被称为"肥沃的土壤"，即有必要的组织支持，以使创新发挥作用并可持续，以及资源的可用性——包括人员、资金、方法论和技能。

加快传播和接受的速度

怎样才能促进更迅速的传播和接受？让我们从历史上选取两个例子：防腐和麻醉。前者的全球传播历时约 30 年，后者为 17 年。如果让患者选择，他们当然会选择两者兼有。为什么会有区别呢？其中一个因素的影响很大，即"对我有什么好处"，还有更多的因素，包括技术、定位的证据，等等。麻醉意味着手术过程中疼痛减轻，但同时也阻止了

less pain during operations but also kept the patient from moving, making the surgeon's life much easier. Antisepsis, by contrast – which initially was a spray of carbolic acid, and the reason for surgeons first using gloves (to protect their skin) – was for the surgeon both unpleasant and hazardous.

Now it would be cynical to suggest that people only adopt that which benefits them. If the benefit is obvious to patients, why would we not use the approach, if, of course, it is easy to implement? As Chip and Dan Heath summarise, to get anyone to change behaviour it is helpful to work through three routes simultaneously seeking emotional buy-in, creating a rational case for change and making the change easy to do (Heath and Heath, 2011). For a further discussion of this topic, including how patients and others may be engaged in change, see Chapter 5.

Once we have thought through an approach under these three broad headings, we have made a good start, but we need to do more. We need a theory of change. Just as we plan a treatment pathway for a patient, we need to plan the introduction of an improvement idea that has worked elsewhere.

Planning for spread and adoption

The first question to ask in planning for spread and adoption is whether the data support the readiness of any approach to be spread; in other words, has it been adequately tested? Just as there are run chart or statistical process control rules about showing the impact of any change, such rules can also help show when an improvement change is sustained and ready to spread. See Chapter 10.

Second, is there capacity and capability to spread the approach? This does not mean using the original person or team repeatedly, unless adequately supported to do so, but determining who has, or needs, capacity and capability to support the implementation in other areas.

Third, have local context and environmental differences from the original site been considered?

Fourth, has some thought been given, not just to what worked in the original site, but also about the pitfalls and how these might be avoided?

患者活动,使外科医生手术时更加轻松。相比之下,防腐剂最初是一种碳酸喷雾,这对外科医生来说既不愉快又危险。这是外科医生使用手套(保护皮肤)的原因。

现在,如果说人们只接受对自己有利的观点,那就太愤世嫉俗了。如果这种方法对患者的益处是显而易见的,那么我们为什么不使用这种方法呢?当然,如果这种方法很容易实现。正如 Chip 和 Dan Heath 总结的那样,要让任何人改变行为,需要通过寻求情感认同、为变革创造合理的理由以及使变革容易实施这 3 种途径来实现(Heath 和 Heath,2011 年)。有关这个主题的更多讨论,包括患者和其他人如何参与变革,请参阅第 5 章。

一旦在这 3 个方面想清楚了方法,我们就有了良好的开端,但是我们需要做更多的事情。我们需要一个变革的理论。正如为患者规划治疗路径一样,我们也需要规划引入一个在其他地方行之有效的改进理念。

为传播和接受做规划

在规划传播和接受时要问的第一个问题是,数据是否随时支持任何手段的传播。换句话说,它是否经过了充分的测试?就像运行图或统计过程控制图可以显示变革的影响一样,此类规则也可以显示维持改进和变革并可以推广的时间。请参阅第 10 章。

第二,这种方法是否有传播的能力?这并不意味着反复使用创始人员或团队,除非得到足够的支持,但要确定谁有能力或需要能力来支持在其他地方的实施。

第三,是否考虑了改进初始地与当地背景和环境差异?

第四,不仅考虑了在改进初始地的工作原理,还考虑了陷阱以及如何避免这些陷阱。

Fifth, are the necessary measurements available and processes for measuring in place (Mountford and Shojania, 2012)?

Finally, it also helps to provide a clear description or design for the work, such as a driver diagram or project plan. People need to understand the approach and thinking of the original work, often across multiple workstreams, and diagrams can be a simple and visual representation to show that. Driver diagrams are described in more detail in Chapter 7.

Practical considerations

Assuming all the above questions have been addressed work can begin, but in seeking to spread effectively, a few practical maxims are worth bearing in mind.

Be tenacious

Not everyone will be ready to make a change at the same time. At any given time, some people will be letting go of the old ways of doing things, others will already be committing to the new, while the majority are in an uncertain, exploratory zone. This requires patience and tenacity in order to move everyone through transition (Bridges 1991). See Box 11.1. The change process is further explored in Chapter 12.

第五，是否有必要的测量方法和适当的测量程序（Mountford 和 Shojania，2012 年）？

最后，使用驱动程序图或项目计划等有助于为工作提供清晰的描述或设计思路。人们需要了解原始工作的方法和思想，通常是跨多个工作流的，而图表可以简单而直观的表示。驱动程序图在第 7 章中有更详细的描述。

实际考虑

假设以上所有问题都已解决，工作就可以开始了，但在寻求有效传播时，有几个实用的准则值得牢记。

坚韧不拔

并非每个人都准备好进行变革。在给定的时间内，有些人将放任旧的做事方式，另一些人将采取新的做事方式，而大多数人则处于不确定性的探索历程。这需要耐心和坚韧，以便使每个人都通过过渡期（Bridges，1991 年）。参见框 11.1。第 12 章将进一步探讨这一变化过程。

Box 11.1 Moving people through transition: an example.
框 11.1　帮人们经历过渡期：一个示例

An improvement team in a large teaching hospital was keen to reap the benefit of patient safety briefings. The aim was to use safety briefings to reduce the level of harm and to spread this to all the wards across the hospital. The approach was an offer of support and evidence of improvement where adopted, but when not welcomed, the team went away for a while and came back when they had more examples of success and tried again. The result was adoption across all appropriate wards over time. Tenacity paid off. The less willing were left alone, and attention focused on those more willing, thus conserving the energy of the team. Eventually, those that had been more sceptical at the start became convinced of the benefits.

一家大型教学医院的改进团队热衷于从患者安全简报中获取信息，其目的是利用安全简报来降低危害程度，并将改进方法传播到全院所有病房。这种方法在采用的病房为其提供支持和改进的证据，但在不受欢迎的时候团队解散了一段时间，当他们有更多成功的例子时又返回来，并再次尝试。结果是随着时间的推移，所有条件合适的病房都采用了这种方法。坚韧得到了回报。不太愿意接受的人被单独留下，注意力集中在那些更愿意接受的人身上，这样就节省了团队的精力。最终，那些在一开始就持怀疑态度的人开始相信这些好处。

Tailor approach to scale

The scale of spread is critical to the approach taken. Spread can mean anything from implementing an improvement in an adjacent similar sized unit, to a national or even international campaign. The larger the adoptive population size, the faster the approach is spread across the population and the smaller the variation in approach across the system. However, very large approaches require significant skill and experience to support, can be very difficult to maintain, overly rigid in their approach and be limited by the ability of very large teams to work effectively together. Improvement approaches and spread have occurred successfully in populations of 2–5 million but less often at larger scale. When planning large scale spread it is important to consider how this may be broken down into smaller subunits, and these matched to the resources at one's disposal.

Provide (some) choice

An ongoing discussion in the literature on dissemination relates to fidelity to the original approach versus local adaptation. Allowing 'a thousand flowers to bloom' can mean there is innovation but also risks introducing unwarranted variation. The balance is difficult but, in general, uniqueness tends to be overemphasised, and around 90% of the context will be similar. So, although some local adaptation of an approach may be necessary, it should not be the other way around.

That said, it is important, in encouraging the implementation of the tried and tested intervention, to recognise the need for a sense of local ownership. One way to achieve this is by creating a fixed aim and level of ambition, with a menu of recommended and tested approaches – not over specified – and to allow each adopting area to pick what is relevant and ignore or adapt what is not.

Patient flow is one area where a lift and drop approach to spread may not work quite so well. There is huge complexity to flow in health systems and the approach taken in one place will not directly translate to another. The principles may be the same, but the relationships, and the part played by different local elements, such as primary care, social services etc., will differ.

量体裁衣

传播的规模依赖于所采取的方法。传播可以意味着任何事情，从邻近的类似规模的单位实施改进，到一个全国性甚至是国际性的运动。接受的群体规模越大，其方法在群体中传播的速度越快，系统中方法的变异就越小。但是，非常复杂的方法需要大量的技能和经验来支持，维护起来非常困难，且方法过于死板，深受大型团队有效协作能力的限制。改进方法及其传播曾在 200 万~500 万人口中取得了成功，但在更大规模下不太常见。当改进计划大规模传播时，重要的是要考虑如何将其分解成更小的子单元，并且这些子单元与可支配的资源相匹配。

提供（一些）选择

传播的文献中涉及对原始方法的忠诚与局部调整之间的关系的讨论。允许"百花齐放"可能意味着创新，但也可能带来不必要的变异。平衡很困难，但总的来说，尽管改进方法大约 90% 是相似的，独特性往往被过分强调。因此，只在有必要时对一种方法进行局部调整，但不应因相似而调整。

也就是说，在鼓励实施久经考验的干预措施时，重要的是要认识到需要有主人翁意识。实现这一目标的一种方法是，建立一个固定的目标和愿景，并提供一份推荐测试方法的清单，而不是过于具体化，并允许每个接受改进方法的地方选择相关的内容，忽略或调整不相关的内容。

患者流使用升降方法进行传播，效果可能不佳。在医疗系统中患者的流动有着巨大的复杂性，在一个地方采取的方法不能直接转化到另一个地方。原则可能是相同的，但不同地方的因素，如初级保健、社会服务等，其关系和作用将有所不同。在这种情况下，人际关系是关键，这显示了在考虑传播和扩

In this situation, relationships are key and this highlights another important point in considering spread and dissemination – who knows who, and can they get on and work together?

Communicate, communicate, communicate

In the internet age, there is no reason not to know what is going on anywhere in the world. Of course, perversely, the availability of so much information overwhelms us, and it is hard to see the wood for the trees. Sometimes when we look for solutions far away, they are in fact available on our door-step. There are many ways to share ideas, projects andlearning and the need for expertise in communications and marketing in quality improvement is often overlooked. The development of the QI Comms Charter by 1000Lives Wales (#QiComms) was a deliberate attempt to address this point (1000 Lives Improvement, 2018).

As outlined in the following section, ideas and knowledge can be shared in many ways but sometimes it is important simply to visit a unit that has adopted a particular approach. You may recall that a similar strategy was advocated in Chapter 6 in relation to identifying a problem. There is much to be gained from this often underused opportunity: seeing an approach in action and learning about any pitfalls and issues in its adoption. Staff involved can also bring life to the benefits both for them and their patients.

Knowledge sharing

Ways to share knowledge include networks, conferences and events and publication in print, virtual print or via social media.

Professional networks

Professional networks in health have existed for years and have shared ideas and approaches. These networks have tended to share new knowledge – a new treatment for cancer, for example – rather than either process approaches or implementation. Specific networks exist now to share improvement knowledge – both physical and virtual and geographically dispersed. The Health Foundations Q Network is one such example which has allowed thousands with an

散时的另一个重要点——谁认识谁，他们能在一起工作吗？

沟通、沟通、沟通

在互联网时代，没有理由不知道世界上任何地方发生了什么。当然，与此相反的是，如此多的信息让我们不知所措，只见树木，不见森林。有时，当我们在遥远的地方寻找解决方案时，它们实际上就在我们的门口。分享想法、项目及学习的方式有很多，而在质量改进方面对传播和营销方面的专业知识的需求常常被忽视。威尔士 1000 场直播（#QiComms）开发的质量改进通讯章程（QI Comms Charter）就是为了解决这一问题（1000 Lives Improvement，2018 年）。

如下一节所述，可以通过多种方式分享想法和知识，但有时只需访问采用特定方法的单位。你可能还记得，在第 6 章中，有人提出了一个类似的策略来发现问题。从这个未被充分利用的机会中，我们可以得到很多好处：看到一种方法正在发挥作用，并了解其采纳过程中出现的任何陷阱和问题。参与的员工也可以为他们自己和患者带来益处。

知识分享

知识共享的方式包括网络、会议和活动以及通过印刷、虚拟印刷或社交媒体进行信息发布。

专业网络

医疗方面的专业网络已经存在多年，并在治疗理论和方法上形成共识。这些网络倾向于共享新知识，例如一种新的癌症治疗方法，而不是共享过程方法或实施方法。现在有了特定的网络来共享改进知识——包括物理的和互联网的，以及被地理所隔绝的知识。健康基金会网络（Health Foundations Q

interest in healthcare improvement to share ideas on both what and how to implement.

Conferences

Conferences can be very energising and sociable, but what part do they play in the spread of ideas (Figure 11.1)? There is now a profusion of quality improvement and patient safety conferences locally, nationally and internationally. What they provide that social media and traditional publications can't is, first, the chance for ideas which may not necessarily be published to be shared. The bar for a poster, for example, is not as high as a talk or peer-reviewed publication. These may be small ideas but may be useful and easily replicated and therefore, if adopted widely, can have a great impact – for example, a safer way of marking pre-operatively or a new way of recording swabs left in situ. Second, they also offer the chance to talk and interact around ideas, to hear from those already doing something and learn from questioning on how an intervention works in practice, creating a dialogue which can be hard to fully experience through reading a publication. Last, improvement ideas presented well can have a real impact on attendees creating time for headspace; many organisations who go as a group 'huddle' daily to share learning and write up their findings for a wider audience in their own place of work.

Network）就是这样一个例子，它让成千上万对医疗保健改进感兴趣的人分享了关于实施什么和如何实施的想法。

会议

会议可以非常活跃和社交化，但是它们在思想传播中扮演什么角色（图 11.1）？目前，在地方、国内和国际上举行了大量的质量改进和患者安全会议。它们提供了什么社交媒体和传统出版物做不到的？首先，可能不一定要发表的想法有了得以分享的机会。例如，海报的门槛不如谈话或同行评议的出版物高。这些想法可能很小，但可能有用，而且易于复制。因此，如果广泛采用，可能会产生很大的影响——例如，一种更安全的术前标记方法或一种新的尚在原地打转的记录拭子方法。其次，他们也提供了一个围绕想法进行交流和互动的机会，听取那些有经验的人的意见，并从提问中学习干预措施在实践中是如何起作用的，创造出一个通过阅读出版物很难完全体验到的对话。最后，精心提出的改进想法可能会给参会人员带来灵感。许多组织每天都"挤作一团"，共同分享学习成果，并在自己的工作场所中为更广泛的受众撰写调查结果。

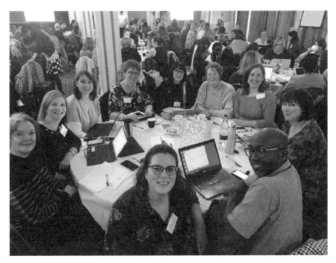

Figure 11.1 Conferences – still relevant in a networked world.
图 11.1　会议在互联网的世界仍然有意义

Publication

Publication still has an important place; the credibility of peer-reviewed work, with statistically proven success, still has a great impact not least for disseminating learning through credible process. Articles appear in a profusion of subject specialist or improvement specialist journals. The need to keep up can seem overwhelming. There are good approaches taken to help any individual in this regard and avoid them missing something relevant. The bulletins of professional bodies (e.g.Royal Colleges) sometimes publish summaries of relevant articles and key word searches of PubMed can keep anyone informed in their areas of interest.

Social media

Social media – such as Twitter, Instagram, Facebook, etc. – is a great way of getting information out there, but promoting and broadcasting news about one's work needs to be planned and worked at in order that key messages rise above the hubbub. Examples are facilitated Twitter-or Facebook-based journal clubs and live webinars. For individuals, as a way of keeping a finger on the pulse it can be extraordinarily effective; but again, it's important to be selective about who to 'follow' in order to distinguish signal from noise. Another key benefit of social media is its ability to forge and build relationships between people who may have never met, sometimes working on opposite sides of the globe.

Conclusion

There is no magic wand for scale up and spread but there are ways of making it easier. Interventions should be tested properly with evidence of impact and be shown to sustain over time. Approaches to dissemination should be planned, easily articulated, clear and consistent, working with the willing early on and the less willing later. Context is all important. Collaboration is more fun than competition and in successful scale up and spread it helps to move to a way of thinking that helps all sides win. Ultimately, of course, our patients and populations must be the beneficiaries.

出版物

出版物仍然占有重要地位。同行评议工作的信誉在统计上证明是成功的，仍然具有很大的影响力，尤其是通过权威学术刊物的传播。文章出现在大量的主题专业期刊或改进专业期刊中。跟上需求的步伐似乎是压倒性的。在这方面，有一些好的方法可以帮助每一个人，避免他们遗漏相关的东西。专业机构（如英国皇家学院）的公告有时会发布相关文章的摘要，PubMed 的关键词搜索可以让所有人都能了解他们感兴趣的领域。

社交媒体

社交媒体如推特、照片墙、脸书等是获取信息的好方法，但发布有关个人工作的信息需要有计划并付出努力，才能使关键信息在喧嚣中凸显。例如基于推特或脸书的期刊俱乐部和现场网络研讨会。对于个人来说，作为一种把握时代脉搏的方法，它可能非常有效；但是，为了区分信号和噪声，有选择地关注是很重要的。社交媒体的另一个关键好处是，它可能让从未谋面的人建立联系，哪怕他们有时工作在地球的两侧。

结论

在扩大宣传规模方面没有魔法棒，但有办法让它更容易。可以对干预措施进行适当的测试，提供能产生影响的证据，并显示其持续时间。传播的方法应该是有计划、易于阐明、明确和一致的，在早期与有意愿的人合作，在后期与不太情愿的人合作。背景非常重要，合作比竞争更有趣。在成功的扩大宣传规模的过程中，合作有助于各方共赢。当然，归根结底，我们的患者和大众必须是受益者。

References
参考文献

1000 Lives Improvement (2018) *QI Comms Charter.* Available at: http://www.1000livesplus.wales.nhs.uk/qicomms (accessed 5 August 2019).

Bridges W. (1991) *Managing Transitions: Making the Most of Change,* Reading, MA, Addison-Wesley.

Dixon-Woods M and Martin G. (2016) Does quality improvement improve quality? *Future Hospital Journal,* 3 (3), 191-194.

Heath C and Heath D. (2011) *Switch: How to Change Things when Change is Hard,* London, Random House.

Morris ZS, Wooding S and Grant J. (2011) The answer is 17 years, what is the question: understanding time lags in translational research. *Journal of the Royal Society of Medicine,* 104 (12), 510-520.

Mountford J and Shojania KG. (2012) Refocusing quality measurement to best support quality improvement: local ownership of quality measurement by clinicians. *BMJ Quality & Safety,* 21 (6), 519-523.

Further reading and resources
深度阅读与相关资源

Massoud MR, Nielsen GA, Nolan K et al. (2006) *A Framework for Spread: From Local Improvements to System-Wide Change,* IHI Innovation Series white paper, Cambridge, MA, Institute for Healthcare Improvement.

McCannon CJ, Schall MW and Perla RJ. (2008) *Planning for Scale: A Guide for Designing Large-Scale Improvement Initiatives,* IHI Innovation Series white paper, Cambridge, MA, Institute for Healthcare Improvement; 2008.

Institute for Healthcare Improvement. Available at: www.ihi.org/ resources/Pages/Tools/IHISevenSpreadlySins.aspx (accessed 5 August 2019).

NHS Scotland Quality Improvement Hub. *The Spread and Sustainability of Quality Improvement in Healthcare.* Available at: www.qihub.scot.nhs.uk/media/596811/the%20spread% 20and%20sustainability%20ofquality%20 improvement% 20in%20healthcare%20pdf%20.pdf (accessed 5 August 2019).

Shaw J, Shaw S, Wherton J. et al. (2017) Studying scale-up and spread as social practice: theoretical introduction and empirical case study. *Journal of Medical Internet Research,* 19 (7), e244.

The Health Foundation (2018) *The Spread Challenge. How to Support the Successful Uptake of Innovations and Improvements in Health Care.* Available at: www.health.org.uk/publications/ the-spread-challenge (accessed 5 August 2019).

第12章 | 理解变革

Brian Marshall

Academic Director, Organisational Development and Change Discipline Lead, Ashridge-Hult, Berkhamsted, UK

OVERVIEW
概述

- How we think about change has, itself, changed.
  我们对变革本身的看法已经改变。
- This parallels changes in society and the expectations of individuals.
  这与社会的变化和个人的期望相类似。
- How we 'do' change has shifted from a starting point of no discussion imposition, through top-down and vision-led change, to more participative approaches which seek to involve those most affected.
  我们如何"制造"变革已经从一个没有讨论价值的起点，通过自上而下和愿景导向的改变，转变为更具参与性的方法，并寻求让受益最多的人参与进来。
- Participative change may be a more successful strategy than simply trying to push change through.
  参与式变革可能是一个比仅仅试图推动变革更成功的策略。

'While all changes do not lead to improvement, all improvement requires change.'
(Institute of Healthcare Improvement, 2019)

The implications of this opening quote are clear; if we want to improve quality in healthcare, we must change something, but just because we've made a change doesn't mean it will necessarily be a change for the better. So, in order to make changes that matter, we need to understand how change itself can be understood. And our understanding and expectations of change have themselves shifted significantly over recent decades. Figure 12.1 provides a simplified view of how some of these shifts have manifested themselves.

For a long period in the early history of organisational life, change was simply a matter of following instructions. Company leaders, often individual business owners, felt it completely within their range of legitimate action to simply enforce whatever changes were deemed

"虽然不是所有的变革都导致改进，但所有的改进都需要变革。"（医疗改进研究所，2019年）

这句开场白的含义很清楚，如果我们想提高医疗质量，则必须改变一些东西，但仅仅因为我们已经做出了变革并不意味着它一定会变得更好。因此，为了做出重要的变革，我们需要理解变革。几十年来，我们对变革的理解和期望也发生了重大变化。图12.1提供了一个简化的视图，展示了其中一些转变是如何表现出来的。

在早期很长一段时间的组织生活中，变革仅仅是遵循指示。公司领导者通常是个体企业主，完全在他们的合法行动范围内，可以简单地执行认为必要的更改。这反映了将组织视为可控机构的观点，除了通过教条法

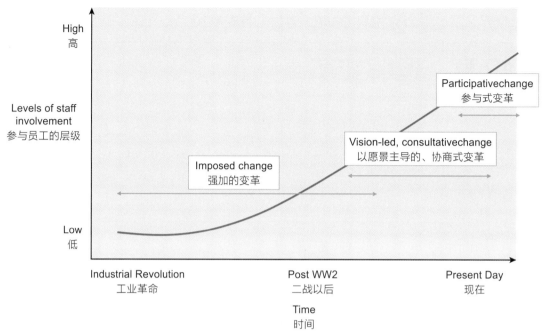

Figure 12.1 The changing face of change.

图 12.1 变革的变迁

necessary. Reflecting a view of organisations as mechanisms to be controlled, it would probably have seemed unusual to doanything other than impose the changes required via dogmatic decree. As the rights and needs of the individual began to receive more emphasis in the Western world – and it is interesting to note how societal attitudes and norms are reflected in organisational approaches – so a reluctance to accept change without personal involvement has grown.

令强制实施所需的变革之外，做任何事情都可能显得不同寻常。随着个人权利和需求在西方世界受到更多的重视——注意到社会态度和规范如何反映在组织方法中也很有趣。因此，人们越来越不愿意接受没有个人参与的变革。

Step-wise, top-down change

逐步、自上而下的变革

There began to be a growing awareness in the 1980s that change did not often happen in the way which had been intended and that much of it just did not stick. There is a much-quoted idea that '70% of change efforts fail', and although the evidence base for that figure is disputed, we have all experienced change which did not achieve its stated objectives, which overran or overspent, or which quickly returned to its original state once senior managers stopped paying attention. Looking to address some of these issues, there emerged a flurry of change methodologies in the 1990s, often steps or processes which offered the prospect

在 20 世纪 80 年代，人们开始越来越意识到，变革并不经常以预期的方式发生，而且很多变革都没有坚持下去。有一种被广泛引用的观点认为 70% 的变革尝试都失败了，尽管这一数字的证据存在争议，但我们都经历过没有实现既定目标的变革，变革太过或花费过多，或者一旦高级管理人员不再关注，变革很快就回到了最初的状态。为了解决其中的一些问题，在 20 世纪 90 年代出现了一系列变革方法，常常采用一些步骤或流

of controlled, successful change. Perhaps the most well-known of these is John Kotter's 8-step change process (see Box 12.1), but there are many similarities between them which can be summarised as:

- Diagnose the problem (sometimes not needed depending on starting point).
- Recruit and engage senior management.
- Design the change.
- Communicate it downwards.
- Embed it.

These types of approaches certainly feel like a step forward in making change happen. They provide a structure which is helpful when we don't know where to begin and take into account the need to ensure that those affected by the change know why it's happening. However, there are a number of difficulties with this kind of approach. First, the implication that change is a relatively orderly process which has a clear scope and starting point, and where it is possible to assess progress at each step. In some rare instances this may the case, but where the change is much messier, treating it in this way can ignore what is really happening and thus lead to change rejection and failure. Second, and perhaps more significantly, is that this process is

程来提供可控、成功的变革前景。其中最著名的可能是约翰·科特的 8 步变革流程（框12.1），但各种流程之间有许多相似之处，可以概括为：

- 诊断问题（有时不需要，具体取决于起点）。
- 招聘并聘请高级管理人员。
- 设计变革。
- 向下沟通。
- 嵌入变革。

这些方法让人感觉在实现变革方面迈出了一步。它们提供了一种框架，当我们不知道从哪里开始，并且需要确保受益的人知道变革发生的原因时，该框架将很有帮助。但是，这种方法存在许多困难。首先，隐含的变革是一个相对有序的过程，具有明确的范围和起点，可以在每个步骤中评估进度。只有在某些罕见的情况下才可能会发生这种情况，但是在变革较为混乱的情况下，以这种方式处理可能会忽略实际发生的事情，从而

Box 12.1 **Leading change. John Kotter's 8-step model.**
框 12.1　**引领变革。约翰·科特的 8 步模式**

- Establishing a sense of urgency.
  建立紧迫感。
- Creating the guiding coalition.
  建立指导联盟。
- Developing a vision and strategy.
  制定愿景和战略。
- Communicating the change vision.
  传播变革愿景。
- Empowering employees for broad-based action.
  赋予员工广泛行动的权利。
- Generating short-term wins.
  创造短期收益。
- Consolidating gains and producing more change.
  巩固成果并产生更多变革。
- Anchoring new approaches in the culture.
  在文化的基础上确立新的方法。

Source: Kotter (1996).
来源：约翰·科特（1996 年）。

largely in the hands of the leaders and managers of organisations. There is an assumption that these steps are carried out by the top of the organisation, presumably because they know best. As Henry Mintzberg (2017) has written about this type of change process:

'... read this again, asking yourself, every step of the way, who does each? The chief. Beyond an inner circle, everyone else is there to pursue the vision, obediently ... Powerful individuals who resist the change effort must be removed. What if they have good reason to resist? Can there be no debate, no discussion?'

The implications here are that change driven from the top often feels like it is being imposed, and if there is no room for discussion or involvement, we may find that those we need to be on board are nowhere to be found at the crucial time.

Vision-led change

As we move on chronologically, the vision of the leader, already mentioned in our step-wise process, begins to be given greater emphasis. In this model of change, there is more consideration of the attitudes and feelings of staff lower down the organisation and a recognition that without engaging with them, change efforts will fail. The need to win over their 'hearts and minds' is a key phrase here: unless people really want it and believe in it, the change goal will be elusive.

In this approach, the winning of the hearts and minds is through the vision of the future painted by the top leaders, usually one leader – the Chief Executive. It falls to him or her to see the bright possibility of a glorious organisational future, and the changes that are necessary to reach this state. Often this kind of vision-led change is accompanied by a strong communication drive, to make sure we have all heard (and hopefully been stirred by) the message from the top. If we have not 'bought in' to the vision it will usually be seen as for one or more of the following reasons: (i) we have not really appreciated the full power of the vision; (ii) we do not understand what's in it for us – employees are seen as basically interested in their own small world and need to

导致变革受阻甚至失败。其次，也许更重要的是，这个过程很大程度被掌握在组织的领导者和管理者手中。可以假设这些步骤是由组织的最高层执行的，大概是因为他们最了解。正如亨利·明茨伯格（2017 年）所写的有关这种类型变革过程的文章所言：

"……再读一遍，问问你自己，每一步都是谁做的？头儿。在一个内部圈子之外，其他人都在那里顺从地追求愿景……努力抵制变革的强人必须被清除。如果他们有好的理由反抗，难道没有辩论，没有讨论吗？"

这里的含义是，高层推动的变革往往让人觉得是强加的，如果没有讨论或参与的空间，我们可能会发现，在关键时刻，我们需要的人无处可寻。

由愿景主导的变革

随着时间的推移，领导者的愿景开始受到更大的重视。在这种变革模式中，需要多考虑底层员工的态度和感受，并意识到如果不与他们合作，变革就会失败。在这里，赢得他们的心是关键：除非人们真的相信他，否则变革的目标将是遥不可及的。

这种方法是通过最高领导者描绘的未来愿景来赢得人心，通常只有一位领导者——首席执行官。他应该看到组织未来的光明前景，以及达到此状态所必需的变革。通常，这种以愿景为导向的变革会伴随着强大的沟通动力，以确保我们都听到了高层传达的信息（且希望被打动）。如果我们不接受这个愿景，通常有以下一个或多个原因：①我们没有真正意识到愿景的全部力量；②我们不明白这对我们有什么好处——员工基本上只对自己的小世界感兴趣，因此需要了解他们将在此变革中所享受到的好处；③我们正在抵抗。

understand the benefits they will enjoy as part of this change; or (iii) we are being resistant.

The solution to each of these perceived problems is the same: explain the vision to people again and again using cascade briefings and town hall meetings, supported with plenty of glossy marketing material – and with increasing volume!

The problem with this approach, again, is two-fold. First, people need to make a transition from where they are currently before they can even consider a significant change. Making this transition is about letting go emotionally of the past, and no amount of recommunication of the vision will help them do that – in fact, it may make them resent the change more. Change is situational and often happens without people transitioning.

Transition is psychological and is a phased process where people gradually accept the details of the new situation and the changes that come with it (see Figure 12.2).

Second, people need to feel that they have a real role in shaping the change and are being treated like adults, with dignity and respect. Most consultation procedures are actually one-way communication processes, where managers avoid awkward questions and employees have no real say or influence.

这些问题的解决方案都是一样的，通过层叠式简报会和员工大会，在大量光鲜亮丽的营销材料的支持下，反复多次向人们解释愿景！

同样，这种方法带来的问题是双重的。首先，人们需要从目前的状况过渡，然后才能考虑重大的变革。做出这种转变意味着在情感上要放弃过去，再多的面对面交流也无助于他们做到这一点——事实上，这可能会让他们更加怨恨这种变革。变革是环境造成的，通常是在人们没有过渡空间的情况下发生的。

过渡是一种心理过程，是一个分阶段的过程，人们逐渐接受新形势的细节和随之而来的变化（图 12.2）。

第二，人们需要感觉到他们在变革过程中扮演了一个货真价实的角色，他们被当作成年人对待，有尊严，被尊重。大多数咨询程序实际上是单向沟通过程，出现管理者逃避尴尬的问题，以及员工没有发言权或影响力的情况。

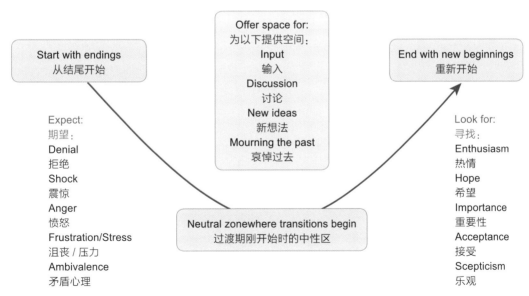

Figure 12.2 Emotional phases of transition. Source: Bridges (2009).

图 12.2　情绪过渡阶段。资料来源：布里奇（2009 年）

Participative change

When the principle of participation is really adopted, it signifies a profound shift in how we think about change. It means a reducing emphasis on planning (reducing our reliance on, say, Gantt charts) and control (a need to ensure that everyone is complying) towards thinking about social and emotional aspects of change.

So how do we approach change and improvement in this way? The first steps are to ensure we know why the improvement is needed, and who we need to involve. Rather than planning out the steps as leader, we begin the change in dialogue with those who enact the process. We frame the issue so that they engage with it and bring their own creativity and experience to making it work. Rather than designing the change and then telling everyone how they must act and feel, the leader's role is to effectivelyframe and communicate the problem, or the question which needs to be answered, in a way which releases energy for those involved. Seeing those affected by the change as the key owners and creators of it, means that the leader's role becomes one which does everything to enable them to fully play that part.

In the process shown in Figure 12.3, the leader seeks to learn as she goes, listening to what is emerging and providing support and input where necessary. Resistance in this model is not seen as unhelpful behaviour, but instead as an indicator that something worthwhile may be being defended, and is therefore worthy of further investigation. In this model, if the change is one which stirs up emotion, then time is allowed for really appreciating what is already working and offering ritual and space to allow people to let go of the past and to move into the future.

Progress is made through experimentation, designing ways of trying things out in order to make sure that whatever change is made will be an improvement – often (but not always) using the Plan Do Study Act (PDSA) cycle.

Often, when the model of participative change is introduced, the reaction is 'I am sure it's a good idea, but I simply don't have time to involve everyone'. This seems at face value to be a reasonable point but it is based on an assumption that top-down change is quick. In

参与式变革

当参与原则真正被接受时，意味着我们对变革的看法发生了深刻的转变。这意味着减少对计划（对甘特图的依赖）和控制（需要确保每个人都遵守）的重视，以考虑在社会和情感方面的变革因素。

那么，我们如何以这种方式对待变革和改进呢？第一步是确保知道为什么需要改进，以及需要让谁参与。我们不是以领导者的身份规划步骤，而是与制定这一进程的人对话。我们制定了这个问题的框架，让他们参与其中，并将自己的创造力和经验带到工作中。领导者的角色不是设计变革，然后告诉每个人必须如何行动和感受，而是有效地构建和传达问题，或者回答问题，从而参与人员赋能。把那些在变革中受到影响的人看作变革的主要拥有者和创造者，意味着领导者变成了一个尽一切努力让他们充分发挥作用的角色。

在图 12.3 所示的过程中，领导者尝试边推进边学，倾听正在出现的情况，并在必要时提供支持，做出投入。对这种模式的抵制并不是无益的行为，而是彰显某些值得捍卫的东西，因此值得进一步研究。在这种模式中，如果变革能够激发情绪的变化，那么就有时间真正地了解已经起作用的事物，并提供仪式和空间，使人们放手过去，走向未来。

进步是通过实验取得的，尝试设计方法，以确保所做的任何变更都是一种进步，经常（但不总是）使用计划 – 执行 – 研究 – 行动（PDSA）循环。

通常，当引入参与式变革模式时，人们的反应是"我确信这是个好主意，但我没有时间让所有人都参与进来"。从表面上看，这似乎是一个合理的观点，但这是基于认为自上而下的变革会很快发生的假设。事实上，宣布变革可能很快，但看到变革的全面实施可能要比让其他人参与变革花费更长的时间。

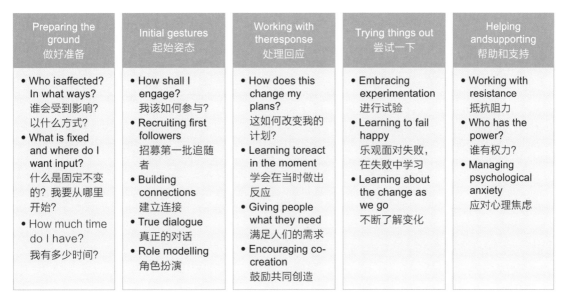

Preparing the ground 做好准备	Initial gestures 起始姿态	Working with theresponse 处理回应	Trying things out 尝试一下	Helping andsupporting 帮助和支持
• Who isaffected? In what ways? 谁会受到影响？以什么方式？ • What is fixed and where do I want input? 什么是固定不变的？我要从哪里开始？ • How much time do I have? 我有多少时间？	• How shall I engage? 我该如何参与？ • Recruiting first followers 招募第一批追随者 • Building connections 建立连接 • True dialogue 真正的对话 • Role modelling 角色扮演	• How does this change my plans? 这如何改变我的计划？ • Learning toreact in the moment 学会在当时做出反应 • Giving people what they need 满足人们的需求 • Encouraging co-creation 鼓励共同创造	• Embracing experimentation 进行试验 • Learning to fail happy 乐观面对失败，在失败中学习 • Learning about the change as we go 不断了解变化	• Working with resistance 抵抗阻力 • Who has the power? 谁有权力？ • Managing psychological anxiety 应对心理焦虑

Figure 12.3 Leading change differently.

图 12.3   引领变革不同的方式

actual fact, announcing change may be quick, but seeing it fully implemented may well take longer than involving others in the change. Participative change can work surprisingly quickly; once folk are engaged, they often move to action without hesitation. Forcing a change can lead to fallout with sometimes disastrous consequences. As Brene Brown (2018) cautions:

'Leaders must either invest a reasonable amount of time attending to fears and feelings or squander an unreasonable amount of time trying to manage ineffective and unproductive behaviour.'

Summary

We began this chapter with the familiar quote: 'While all changes do not lead to improvement, all improvement requires change.' If change is required, we have choices about how we enact that change. While top - down linear change approaches seem appealing because of their clarity, they may lead to active or passive resistance and our improvement initiative will likely run into the ground. Involving people from the outset in shaping the change and allowing the plan to emerge leads to improvement which is shaped and owned by the frontline workers who enact it.

参与式变革的速度惊人地快，一旦人们参与进来，他们往往毫不犹豫地采取行动。强迫改变可能会导致恶果，有时会带来灾难性的后果。正如布雷恩·布朗（2018 年）所警告的：

"领导者要么投入合理的时间关注恐惧和其他感受，要么浪费不合理的时间试图管理无效的行为。"

总结

我们在这一章的开头引用了一句熟悉的话："虽然不是所有的变革都导致改进，但所有的改进都需要变革。"如果需要变革，我们可以选择如何实施这个变革。尽管自上而下的线性变革方法因其清晰性而显得很有吸引力，但它们可能会导致主动或被动的阻力，我们的改进计划可能会付诸东流。从一开始就让人们参与到变革，并允许改进计划的出现，而改进是由制订计划的一线员工推进和拥有的。

References
参考文献

Bridges W. (2009) *Managing Transitions: Making the Most of Change,* 3 edn, London, Nicholas Brealey.

Brown B. (2018) *Dare to Lead: Brave Work. Tough Conversations. Whole Hearts,* London, Vermillion.

Institute for Healthcare Improvement (2019) *Changes for Improvement.* Available at: www.ihi.org/resources/ Pages/ Changes/default.aspx (accessed 5 February 2019).

Kotter J. (1996) *Leading Change,* Brighton, MA, Harvard Business School Publishing.

Mintzberg H. (2017) *Transformation from the Top? How About Engagement on the Ground?* Available at: www. mintzberg.org/ blog/transformation-from-the-top-how-about-engagement-on-the-ground (accessed 14 January 2019).

Further reading and resources
深度阅读与相关资源

Bushe G. (2018) *Generative Leadership.* Unpublished article submitted to the *Canadian Journal of Physician Leadership.* Available at: www.gervasebushe.ca/Generative_Leadership.pdf (accessed 31 January 2019).

Day A. (2011) *Changing the Social Fabric of Organisations: The Importance of Participation.* Available at: https://eoeleadership. hee.nhs.uk/sites/default/files/1317116794_wmbF_changing_ the_social_fabric_of_ organisations.pdf (accessed 15 January 2019).

Holman P, Devane T and Cady S. (ed.) (2017) *The Change Handbook: The Definitive Resource on Today's Best Methods for Engaging Whole Systems,* Oakland, CA, Berrett Koehler.

第13章 | 建立改进文化

Kiran Chauhan

Senior Consultant, Leadership and Organisational Development, The King's Fund, London, UK

OVER VIEW
概述

- Culture can be thought of as the more enduring patterns in what people say, do, think and feel as they try to work together. Perspectives on what those patterns are like will vary across individuals and groups within an organisation.
  文化是人们做集体工作时创造的有利于长期交流、行动、思考、感受的模式。对这些模式的看法将因组织中的个人和团体而异。

- A shared focus on improvement is associated with the delivery of better clinical care in healthcare organisations.
  对改进的普遍关注与医疗机构提供更好的临床护理有关。

- Organisations prioritising improvement will demonstrate that inclusive and purposeful participative learning is important to them, and leaders will role-model these values.
  优先考虑改进的组织将证明，包容性和有目的性的参与式学习对他们来说很重要，领导者将为这些价值观树立榜样。

- Approaches to developing improvement capability can involve a blend of classroom-based learning, coaching and mentoring, and learning through improvement projects.
  发展改进能力的方法包括课堂学习、辅导和指导以及通过改进项目进行学习。

- Everyone in an organisation should be involved in improvement both to demonstrate commitment and to build momentum, though the 'dose' of training required will differ from role to role.
  组织中的每个人都应该参与改进，以展示承诺和建立动力，尽管所需培训的"剂量"因角色而异。

- Positional leaders have a key part to play in setting cultural expectations.
  领导者在设定目标文化方面发挥着关键作用。

What is culture?

什么是文化？

Definitions of organisational culture often tend to take the form of general statements like 'the way we do things around here'. This is partly because what people mean by culture can embrace so many different aspects of the experiences people have of being at work. One way we can be more pragmatic is to see culture as the more enduring patterns in what people say, do, think and feel as they try to work together. These patterns will emerge from what may be very different experiences, some may be

对组织文化的定义通常倾向于采用一般性陈述的形式，比如"我们在这里做事的方式"。这在一定程度上是因为人们所说的文化可以包含工作经历的许多不同方面。更务实的一种方式是，将文化视为人们做集体工作时创造的有利于长期交流、行动、思考、感受的模式。这些模式将出现在非常不同的经历中，一些可能比其他更明显，并且它们可

more noticeable than others, and they are likely to evolve over time. Important interconnected factors to consider are:

- **Perspective:** Each person's experience of their working life is uniquely informed by their background, history and experience. This means there are likely to be as many perspectives of an organisation's culture as there are people.
- **Relationships:** People rarely do their work alone, depending on each other for expertise, resources and support. Processes involving social norms and power relations are inherent in how people work together, but rarely made explicit or talked about openly.
- **Environment:** People joining and leaving teams, and newtechnologies, leaders, policies or governments, can all mean that the circumstances in which people work change frequently. This means that patterns are changing all the time in ways and at speeds we may not expect or notice.

All of these factors make exploring and influencing organisational culture a complex task.

Models of culture

Models that try to articulate what culture is can be useful vehicles for exploring different aspects of organisational life. Cultural models tend to come from the field of organisational development or 'OD' and Figures 13.1 and 13.2 illustrate two examples in common use. Loftus et al. (2015) provide a compendium of models and approaches that may be of interest for further reading.

Models of organisational culture can help to inform decisions about how to influence ways of working; however, the temptation to rely on them as definitive accounts of people's experience should be resisted: as the statistician George Box wrote, 'all models are wrong, but some are useful' (1979). So, rather than seeing them as just diagnostic tools, models should always be considered for their usefulness in context and as a part of the process of change.

For example, in an organisation where conflict seems to be an ongoing issue in getting improvement off the ground, Schein's iceberg model (1992) may help people to explore the rarely discussed assumptions which may underlie this conflict. Or in an organisation that

能会随着时间的推移而演变。需要考虑的重要因素包括：

- **视角：** 每个人的工作经历都有其独特的背景、历史和经验。这意味着组织的文化前景可能和个人的一样多。
- **人际关系：** 人们很少单独工作，依赖彼此的专业知识、资源和支持。涉及社会规范和权力关系的过程是集体工作的固有过程，但很少被明确或公开谈论。
- **环境：** 人们加入或离开团队，新的技术、领导者、政策或政府都可能意味着工作环境发生变化。这意味着文化模式一直在以我们无法预料或注意到的方式和速度变化着。

所有这些因素使得探索和影响组织文化成为一项复杂的任务。

文化模式

试图阐明什么是文化模式可以把它变成探索组织生活不同方面的有用工具。文化模式往往来自组织发展领域，图 13.1 和 13.2 说明了两个常用的例子。洛夫图斯等（2015 年）提供了一份模式和方法概要，供进一步阅读。

组织文化模式可以说明决策是如何影响工作方式的；然而，应该抵制将这些模式作为替代人们经验的诱惑。正如统计学家乔治·博克斯所写的，"所有模式都错了，但有些模式是有用的"（1979 年）。因此，不应将模式仅仅视为诊断工具，而应始终考虑模式在背景中及作为变革流程一部分的有效性。

例如，在一个组织中，冲突似乎是改进道路上的一个持续的问题，沙因的"冰山模型"（1992 年）能够帮助人们探索可能引起冲突的那些鲜为人知的假设。或者，对于一个似乎非常依赖控制系统和组织结构来创造改进热情的组织，约翰逊和斯科尔斯的文化网络（2009 年）可能会帮助人们将注意力转

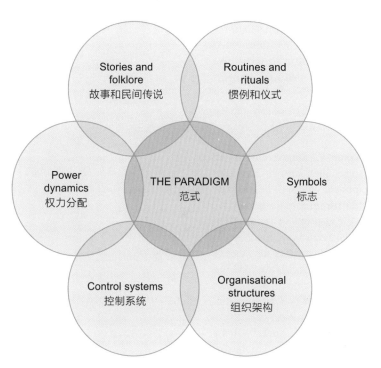

Figure 13.1 Cultural web. Source: Adapted from Johnson et al. (2009).

图 **13.1** 文化网络。资料来源：改编自约翰逊等（2009 年）

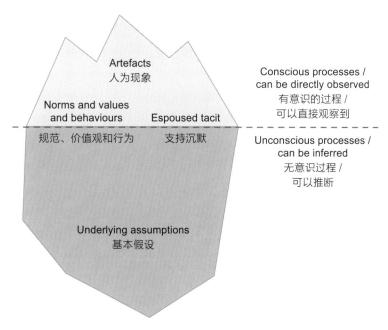

Figure 13.2 Cultural iceberg. Source: Adapted from Schein (1992).

图 **13.2** 文化冰山。资料来源：改编自沙因（1992 年）

seems to rely heavily on control systems and organisational structures to create enthusiasm for improvement, Johnson and Scholes' cultural web (2009) may help to draw attention to what else could be done, beyond people's natural comfort zones.

Cultures of improvement

As described in Chapter 12, improvement can be thought of as changes that lead to learning, usually involving the people who will be affected by the change. In healthcare organisations, this is likely to be in the context of the quality, experience and cost-effectiveness of the clinical services that patients, their families and carers receive, and there is growing evidence linking organisational focus on improvement with better healthcare delivery (Care Quality Commission, 2018). Using the working definition of culture provided earlier, improvement cultures will be manifest as patterns of interaction that emphasise the importance of participative learning in moving towards these goals.

The more that people are learning about improvement, and working on improvement projects, the more likely it will be to become a pattern in the organisation that can be described as an improvement culture. These kinds of change processes tend to involve trying to reach a critical mass where the change effort becomes more self - sustaining, encouraged by people starting to see service outcomes changing sustainably because of their improvement work, or their work being celebrated, or support mechanisms being established to enable further improvement work.

Building improvement capacity and capability

There is little research available comparing the effectiveness of different approaches to learning about improvement (The Health Foundation, 2012). Didactic, social and 'on the job' learning experiences are all thought to be important aspects of education and training programmes, but none is likely to be sufficient on its own. Lombardo and Eichinger (1996) are known for the introducing the now widely used '70:20:10' learning and development model (Figure 13.3).

移到舒适区之外的其他事情上。

改进文化

如第 12 章所述，改进能导致学习方式的变革，通常涉及受到变革影响的人。在医疗机构中，这可能与患者、家属和护理人员所接受的临床服务质量、体验和成本效益有关，越来越多的证据表明，组织对改进的关注与更好的医疗服务是相关联的（医疗质量委员会，2018 年）。使用前面给出的关于工作文化的定义，改进文化将表现为互动模式，强调参与式学习在实现这些目标中的重要性。

人们对改进的了解越多，越投入到改进项目中，就越有可能形成一种组织中可以称为改进文化的模式。这些类型的变革流程往往试图达到某个临界质量水平，在这个临界质量水平上，变革工作可以自我维持，人们开始看到服务结果因其改进工作或其工作受到赞扬而持续改变，或建立支持机制，以便进一步参与改进工作。

培育改进能力

关于学习改进的各种方法，很少研究比较其有效性（健康基金会，2012 年）。说教、社交和在职学习经历都被认为是教育和培训方案的重要方面，但仅凭这些经验是不够的。隆巴多和艾辛格（1996 年）以引入目前广泛使用的 "70：20：10" 学习和发展模式而闻名（图 13.3）。

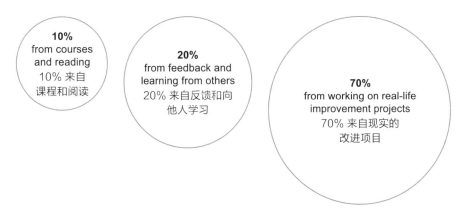

Figure 13.3 The 70 : 20 : 10 principle. Source: Adapted from Lombardo and Eichinger (1996).

图 13.3　70∶20∶10 原理。资料来源：改编自隆巴多和艾辛格（1996 年）

They suggest:

'Development generally begins with a realization of current or future need and the motivation to do something about it. This might come from feedback, a mistake, watching other people's reactions, failing or not being up to a task – in other words, from experience.'

Previous education or training experiences, and the local context, will all influence what kinds of encounters will trigger learning processes for different people. Particularly because approaches to learning are diversifying as new technologies become available, one size is unlikely to fit all. One way of appealing to a range of preferences, particularly when multiprofessional teams are undertaking training together, is to use blended approaches that enable learners to engage in ways that suit them. It is important to remember that people often stay in their comfort zones, so approaches should encourage individuals and teams to experiment with new ways of thinking. In addition, providing time to reflect on how they are finding the learning process, and how they might improve it, is a further opportunity to develop improvement or innovation capacity (Edmondson, 2014).

The impact of these approaches can be enhanced over time by defining the intended outcomes of improvement training and measuring whether these are being achieved using the methodologies described in previous

他们建议：

"发展通常始于对当前或未来需求的认识以及为此采取行动的动力。这可能来自反馈、失误、观察别人的反应、失败或不能胜任某项任务——换言之，来自经验。"

以前的教育或培训经历，以及当地的环境，对于什么样的遭遇会触发人的学习过程都会产生影响。特别是由于学习方法随着新技术的出现而多样化，同一尺度不可能适合所有人。吸引多样人群的一种办法是使用混合方法，让学习者以适合他们的方式参与其中，特别是在多专业团队接受培训时。重要的是，要记住人们往往停留在自己的舒适区，因此应该鼓励个人和团队尝试新的思维方式。此外，花时间思考如何找到适当的学习过程以及如何改进它，这是进一步发展改进或创新能力的机会（Edmondson，2014 年）。

随着时间的推移，通过定义改进培训的预期结果，并通过使用前几章中描述的方法来衡量是否实现了这些目标，可以提高这些方法的影响力。作为组织控制系统的一部分，监控进度并相应地调整培训过程可以为进一步提高组织在改进工作中的形象提供方法，这也有助于人们理解改进的核心概念。

chapters. Monitoring progress and adjusting the training process accordingly as part of the organisation's control systems can provide further ways to raise the profile of improvement work the organisation, which also helps people to understand core improvement concepts.

Importantly, not everyone needs to know everything about improvement for it to thrive within an organisation. The Academy of Medical Royal Colleges (2016) have drawn the parallel with cardio - pulmonary resuscitation (CPR). CPR training is universal for health workers, easily learnt and experienced through simulation and experiential learning, usually working as a multiprofessional team. Even if not performing CPR, the basic principles can be understood and any worker may be called upon to help if needed. Building on this, the concept of 'dosing' introduced by Lloyd (2017) is a helpful way to think about how people's training needs will differ from role to role. Just as the appropriate dose of a medicine may be higher or lower from patient to patient due to age, body weight or what other medications they are taking, for improvement, contextual factors should inform the approach taken. The size of the organisation, who is formally and informally influential, or what other change initiatives are also going on, may all be important in determining what 'dose' of improvement knowledge and experience is appropriate for people with different roles.

The table in Box 13.1 below indicates some of the priorities at different levels of an organisation, but these need to be tailored to the perspectives, relationships and environments of the specific groups involved, monitored for impact and adjusted according to how patterns start to change. Building an improvement culture therefore cannot be a 'do once' activity; instead, it needs to be an ongoing, iterative learning process involving people at all levels of organisations, which itself models the principles of improvement.

Leading an improvement culture

Twenty-first-century healthcare is increasingly delivered by wide networks of organisations working together to provide services to large populations. A typical hospital team may be working at any given time with community health teams, general practitioners, social care

重要的是，并不是每个人都需要了解关于改进的所有知识才能让它在组织中蓬勃发展。英国皇家医学院（2016 年）已将其与心肺复苏（CPR）相提并论。CPR 培训对于医疗工作者来说比较普遍，通常需要多专业团队合作，可以通过模拟和体验式学习轻松地学习和体验。即使不执行心肺复苏，也可以理解基本原理，如有需要，可以为任何人提供帮助。在此基础上，劳埃德（2017 年）提出的"剂量"概念是考虑到人们的培训需求因角色而异。正如由于年龄、体重或他们正在服用其他药物，不同患者的药物剂量可能不同，为了改善效果，应结合背景因素来决定所采用的方法。组织的规模，谁正式或非正式地有影响，或者有其他正在进行的变革举措，确定不同角色的人适合什么"剂量"的改进知识和经验很重要。

下面的框 13.1 中的表格显示了一个组织不同级别的优先事项，但这些优先事项需要根据所涉群体的视角、关系和环境进行调整，监测影响，并根据模式的变化进行调整。因此，建立改进文化不是"一次性"活动，而是需要一个持续的、迭代的学习过程，涉及组织各个层面的人员，这本身就是改进原则的模式。

领导改进文化

21 世纪的医疗保健越来越多地通过大型的组织网络提供，这些组织共同为广大人群提供服务。一个典型的医院团队可能在任何给定的时间与社区医疗团队、全科医生、社

Box 13.1 **Improvement knowledge and activities.**
框 13.1　**改进知识和改进活动**

Who 谁	What do they need to know? 他们需要知道什么	What do they need to do? 他们需要做什么
Frontline staff 一线员工	• key improvement concepts 主要的改进理念	• identify improvement opportunities 识别改进的机会 • contribute to or lead local projects 参与或领导当地的项目
Managers 管理者	• key improvement concepts 主要的改进理念 • local improvement methodology 当地的改进方法	• manage improvement projects 管理改进项目 • enable participation 促成员工参与改进 • coach and mentor 教练和导师
Senior leaders 高级领导者	• key improvement concepts 主要的改进理念 • tools relevant to leading for improvement 与领导改进相关的工具	• set direction 确定方向 • emphasise importance of improvement 强调改进的重要性 • ensure improvement 确保改进的进行
Experts 专家	• deep knowledge of improvement theory 精通改进理论 • extensive practical experience 丰富的实践经验	• provide support, advice and training 提供支持、建议和培训 • coach and mentor 教练和导师

services and local authorities, sometimes in ways they aren't immediately aware of. They will also be relying on suppliers of clinical consumables, medicines, waste disposal and a range of other services. All these other parties will influence what happens in the organisation in small ways, and when we start to appreciate the huge numbers of people who are therefore directly and indirectly involved with the business of delivery, it becomes clear why trying to realise intended changes can be difficult.

Acknowledging this changing context, recent research has emphasised the need for distributed forms of leadership in contrast to the 'command and control' approaches that have been prevalent in the past (West et al., 2015). This move away from some of the principles of traditional 'top down' management can also be seen as a recognition of how difficult it is for formal leaders to control what happens in their organisations, especially when those organisations are particularly large or complex, or their operating environment is in flux.

会护理服务机构以及地方当局合作，有时他们可能并没有立即意识到。他们还将依赖临床耗材、药品、废物处理和一系列其他服务的供应商。这些方面都会以微小的方式影响组织中发生的事情，当我们开始意识到有大量的人因此直接或间接参与到业务交付，我们就会明白为什么实现预期的变革是困难的。

认识到这种不断变化的背景后，最近有研究强调了与过去流行的"指挥和控制"方法相比，分布式领导形式的必要性（West 等，2015 年）。这种背离传统的自上而下管理原则的做法，也可以视为领导者意识到，要控制其组织中发生的事情是多么困难，尤其是当这些组织特别庞大复杂，或其经营环境不断变化时。

While culture may not be in the gift of any one person to control, formal, or positional, leaders are important because they can do things that most others cannot. This may include rewarding certain activities and sanctioning others; or allocating resources in one area and not in another; or engaging with some people and not with others. While their directions may not always be followed as they would like, leaders can still influence what others do in significant ways; what they say, do and pay attention to can set the tone for the rest of the organisation. Leaders at all levels may find it useful to consider the questions in Figure 13.4 to explore how their own behaviours might be part of what seems to be working well, and less well, in their organisations.

Leaders can support cultures of improvement, specifically, by ensuring that the principles discussed above are reflected in all aspects of how their organisations work. Applying the cultural web, Box 13.2 gives examples of patterns that might indicate that improvement is important and, using the iceberg model, what assumptions might be involved in those patterns. Leaders at all levels can demonstrate these priorities through their own behaviour and, consistent with the principles of improvement science, they can iteratively experiment with changes to their approaches, using their learning to inform future actions.

虽然文化不是某个人天生就能够控制的，但无论是对于正式的还是职位上的领导者都很重要，因为他们能做大多数人做不到的事情。这包括奖励和惩罚；或者为某个领域注入资源；或者与某些人而不是与其他人交往。虽然方向可能并不总是如他们所愿，但领导者仍然可以以重要的方式影响他人的行为；他们所说、所做和所关注的可以为组织的其他成员定下基调。各级领导可能会发现考虑图 13.4 中的问题是很有益的，能够探索他们自己的行为如何成为组织中运作良好或不太良好的一部分。

领导者支持改进文化，具体来说，就是确保上述原则反映在组织工作的各个方面。框 13.2 运用文化网络，举例说明了一些模式，这些模式表明改进很重要，再使用冰山模型，可以分析这些模式可能涉及哪些假设。各级领导都可以通过自己的行为来论证这些优先事项，并且按照改进的科学原则，他们可以反复尝试改变他们的方法，利用他们的学习成果来指导未来的行动。

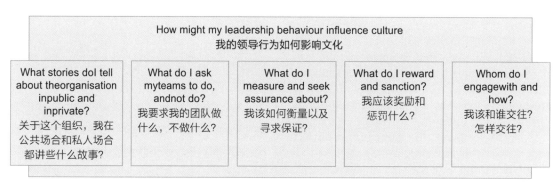

Figure 13.4 How can leadership behaviour influence culture?

图 13.4　领导行为如何影响文化

Box 13.2 **Patterns and assumptions in cultures of improvement.**
框 13.2 **改进文化的模式和假设**

Cultural web element 组成文化的元素	Examples of patterns you might see 可能看到的模式示例	What assumptions could be implied? 可能隐含哪些假设
Stories and folklore 故事和民间传说	• People at all levels talk readily about their improvement work, what is working, what isn't, and what they're learning 所有级别的人都乐于谈论改进工作，什么有效，什么无效，以及他们正在学习什么 • Key organisational successes are framed through an improvement lens 组织的关键成功是通过改进的视角构建的 • Improvers and their achievements are well-known and regarded 改进者的成就众所周知	• Improvement and learning are valued, both in behaviour and resources 改进和学习在行为和资源方面都很重要 • Things not going to plan are opportunities to learn 没有按计划发生的事是学习的机会 • Everyone should be able to access training and development easily, and have time to take these up 每个人都有时间轻松地获得培训和发展 • Helping others to learn is as important as individual learning 帮助他人学习和自己学习同样重要 • Diversity leads to better improvement work 多样性会让改进工作更好 • Everyone's contributions are valued regardless of specific roles. 无论具体角色如何，每个人的付出都是有价值的
Rituals and routines 仪式和惯例	• People are using improvement tools to experiment and learn all the time 人们一直在使用改进工具进行试验和学习 • Improvement features in the organisation's formal rituals, for example staff awards, annual general meetings, or recruitment processes 组织中正式仪式如员工奖励、年度股东大会或招聘流程的改进	
Symbols 标志	• People wear badges or clothing that denote levels of improvement experience, expertise, or availability to support others 人们佩戴徽章或穿着特殊服装，表示有经验、专业知识或支持他人改进的能力 • Visual artefacts showcase improvement projects, the use of improvement tools, or opportunities to get involved in improvement work across the organization 改进项目可视化和改进工具的使用可以让整个组织都改进工作参与	
Organisational structures 组织结构	• Resources are allocated to supporting improvement, including training and development 分配资源用于支持改进，包括培训和发展 • There are people in senior improvement roles in the organisation who champion the work internally and externally 组织中有一些担任高级改进角色的人，他们在内部和外部都支持这项工作	
Control systems 控制系统	• Progress on improvement projects features on meeting agendas from the boardroom to 'frontline' teams 从董事会到一线团队会议议程的改进项目进展情况 • Time-series data are used for measuring improvement and to inform decision-making 时间线数据用于测量改进情况并为决策提供信息 • Recruitment criteria include improvement skills and experience 招聘标准包括改进技能和经验 • Doing improvement work features in appraisal and performance frameworks 在评估和绩效框架中进行改进工作 • Training courses and support systems for improvement work are easy to find and access 培训课程和改进工作的支持系统很容易找到和使用	
Power dynamics 权力分配	• People doing improvement have influence in the organisation; their voices are heard at all levels 从事改进工作的人在组织中有影响力，他们的声音让各个层次的人都能听到 • Hierarchy seems less important than the ability contribute 等级制度似乎不如能力输出那么重要 • People with diverse backgrounds are involved in improvement work 让不同背景的人都参与到改进工作中	

Summary

The context and culture in which improvement activities take place will heavily influence their success and sustainability. Not everyone needs to know everything about improvement for it to thrive within an organisation, but building capability in a contextually appropriate way is at the heart. Leadership then plays a critical role in influencing connectedness of relationships and how they are strengthened as improvement capacity is built.

总结

进行改进活动的环境和文化将严重影响其成功和可持续性。并非每个人都需要了解有关改进的所有知识以使其在组织中蓬勃发展，但是以适合背景的方式进行能力建设是其核心。此外，领导力在打通人际关系以及建立改进能力时如何加强这些关系至关重要。

References
参考文献

Academy of Medical Royal Colleges (2016) *Training for Better Outcomes,* London, Academy of Medical Royal Colleges. Available at: https://www.aomrc.org.uk/wp-content/uploads/ 2016/06/Quality_improvement_key_findings_140316-2.pdf. (accessed 15 May 2019).

Box GEP. (1979) Robustness in the strategy of scientific model building, in *Robustness in Statistics* (ed. RL Launer and GN Wilkinson), Cambridge, MA, Academic Press, 201-236.

Care Quality Commission (2018) *Quality Improvement in Hospital Trusts. Sharing Learning from Trusts on a Journey of QI.* Availableat: https://www.cqc.org.uk/publications/evaluation/quality-improvement-hospital-trusts-sharing-learning-trusts-journey-qi (accessed 12 March 2019).

Edmondson AC. (2014) *Teaming to Innovate,* San Francisco, Jossey-Bass.

Johnson G, Scholes K and Whittington R (2009) *Fundamentals of Strategy,* Harlow, Pearson Education.

Lloyd R. (2017) *Quality Health Care: A Guide to Developing and Using Indicators,* 2nd edn, Burlington, MA, Jones & Bartlett Learning.

Lombardo M and Eichinger RW. (1996) *The Career Architect Development Planner,* Minneapolis, Lominger.

Schein E. (1992) *Organizational Culture and Leadership,* San Francisco, Jossey Bass.

The Health Foundation (2012) *Quality Improvement Training for Healthcare Professionals.* Available at: https:// www.health.org. uk/publications/quality-improvement-training-for-healthcare-professionals (accessed 12 March 2019).

West M, Armit K, Loewenthal L et al. (2015) *Leadership and Leadership Development in Healthcare: The Evidence Base,* London, The King's Fund.

Further reading and resources
深度阅读与相关资源

Loftus E, Jarvis J and Atkinson J. (2015) *The Art of Change Making.* Available at: www.leadershipcentre.org.uk/wp-content/ uploads/2016/02/The-Art-of-Change-Making.pdf (accessed 12 March 2019).

NHS Improvement (2017) *Building Capacity and Capability for Improvement: Embedding Quality Improvement Skills in NHS Providers.* Available at: https://improvement.nhs.uk/ documents/1660/01-NHS107-Dosing_Document-010917_K_1. pdf (accessed 12 March 2019).

Stacey RD. (2012) *Tools and Techniques of Leadership and Management: Meeting the Challenge of Complexity,* London, Routledge.

第14章 | 质量改进的未来

Emma Vaux[1] and Tim Swanwick[2]

[1] Consultant nephrologist and general physician, Royal Berkshire NHS Foundation Trust; Vice President for Education and Training, Royal College of Physicians (RCP), London, UK

[2] Director, Clinical Leadership Development, NHS Leadership Academy, NHS England and NHS Improvement, Leeds, UK

OVER VIEW
概述

- With the arrival of the 'fourth industrial revolution', medicine is being reimagined.
  随着第四次工业革命的到来，医学正在被重新构想。

- The ability to respond to, influence and shape this rapid era of change is essential.
  应对、影响和塑造这个快速变化时代的能力至关重要。

- Advances in technology bring new ways of obtaining and using data for continuous learning and improvement.
  技术进步带来了获取和使用数据的新方法，以持续学习和改进。

- An individual's experience of implementing change within a microsystem should be aligned with whole systems thinking and learning for effective improvement change.
  个人在小型系统内实施变革的经验应与整个系统的思考和学习保持一致，以有效地改进变革。

- Quality improvement capability has a significant role to play in delivering a sustainable future for health and healthcare.
  质量改进能力在为健康和医疗提供可持续未来方面发挥着重要作用。

The fourth industrial revolution

'The fourth industrial revolution is here.' (World Economic Forum, 2019)

The first industrial revolution brought mechanisation, waterpower and steam; the second, the application of science to mass production; and the third, computerisation and automation. The fourth industrial revolution brings cyber-physical systems and heralds profound change across many sectors and aspects of human life in how we deliver, and how patients consume, health and healthcare. The ability to leverage artificial intelligence (AI), big data and smart analytics, virtual and augmented reality, nanotechnologies and modern machines

第四次工业革命

"第四次工业革命已经到来。"（世界经济论坛，2019 年）

第一次工业革命带来了机械化、水力和蒸汽机；第二次工业革命，科学在大规模生产中得到应用；第三次工业革命为计算机和自动化。第四次工业革命带来了物联网，预示着人类生活的许多领域发生了深刻的变化，包括我们如何提供服务、患者如何享受健康和医疗保健服务。利用人工智能（AI）、大数据和智能分析、虚拟现实和增强现实、纳

(robotics, drones, 3D-printing) is changing prevailing healthcare models to personalised continuums of care with a greater focus on prevention and early intervention. It is an era of people power and social and technological connectedness of communities facilitated by emerging digital technologies.

In such a period of relentless and rapid change, never has it been more relevant to learn skills in quality improvement in order to play an effective role in the world. AI and machine learning will increasingly surface and question areas of our professional practice as we experience continuous quality improvement in action. We will need to be comfortable and experienced in challenging and critiquing different models, and their risks, and encourage and support others to develop and design clinically appropriate and person - centric solutions.

Implications for healthcare improvement

Utilisation of data

Quality improvement starts with understanding a problem and then understanding the impact of any change; how we use and manipulate data to inform these processes is of central importance.

Emerging technology is providing us with the ability to extract data in new and innovative ways; continuously, remotely, on the move. This accelerates an existing trend towards person-centric models of health and care, shifting the locus of care away from the acute hospital to the community and the home. To maximise value we will need to understand the ways in which data is collected and filtered, and how digital outputs can be deployed with proper consideration to clinical, social and ethical context. Used wisely, technology will create time for higher level activities with more emphasis on the value of high-quality decision making, notably concerning the managing of uncertainty and risk in the digital world. Ensuring that we pose the right questions and are able to respond to, lead and implement improvement in an environment where data are so readily available – and in such vast quantities – becomes ever more important.

Technology also enables us to share data more effectively and inincreasingly sophisticated

米技术和现代机器（机器人、无人机、3D打印）的使用正在改变主流的医疗模式，使之成为个性化的连续护理模式，更加注重预防和早期干预。这是一个由新兴数字技术推动的人力、社会与社区技术联通的时代。

在这个日新月异的时代，学习质量改进技能以希冀为世界做出贡献从来没有像现在这样重要。随着质量改进的持续开展，人工智能和机器学习将不断浮出水面并质疑我们的专业实践。我们需要适应并从容应对挑战和批判不同的模式及其风险，并鼓励、支持其他人开发和设计适合临床并以人为本的解决方案。

医疗改进的意义

数据的利用

质量改进始于了解问题，然后了解变革带来的影响。我们如何使用和分析数据来设计这些流程是至关重要的。

新兴技术为我们提供了以崭新的方式提取数据的能力，能够在变化中持续改进。这加速了现有的以人为本的健康和护理模式的趋势，将护理重心从医院转移到社区和家庭。为了使价值最大化，我们需要了解收集和过滤数据的方式，以及在临床、社会和伦理背景下如何输出数据。如果使用得当，技术将为更高层次的活动创造时间，更加强调高质量决策的价值，特别是关于数字世界中不确定性和风险的管理。提出正确的问题，并能够在数据如此容易获得且数量如此庞大的环境中应对、领导和实施改进，变得越来越重要。

技术还使我们能够以越来越复杂的方式更有效地共享数据。正如人们对大数据的集体意识日益增强，并有可能采用众包解决方案一样，质量改进也应被视为一种集体努力，

ways. In the same way that there is a growing collective mind on big data and a potential to crowd-source solutions, quality improvement should also be seen as a collective endeavour with a focus on communication, teamwork and communities of networks.

Looking further ahead, the promise of AI sees the embedding of continual improvement in automated processes; machines and systems capable of self-development and continual improvement. The role of the quality improver then changes, requiring a whole new set of relationships with those designing AI-led systems, a deep understanding of the decision-making processes and algorithms that lie at their heart and an oversight function ensuring that all change, however initiated, is an improvement.

Systems thinking

Any improvement initiative requires us to consider how to integrate our efforts with daily clinical operations and professional development. Ideally, the aim is to have coordinated, evaluated, large-scale efforts to improve fidelity of practice across systems of care. This involves thinking in terms of systems, technologies and processes, many of which are interconnected making the context of any improvement effort complex.

By using a systems approach the intention is to deter mine the system design and implementation strategy that delivers the best service (Royal Academy of Engineering, 2017). Existing improvement approaches may be enhanced by using techniques from system engineering in tandem. These include inclusive design which asks the important questions: 'what proportion of our service users can easily access the service we offer; and how do we systematically design for maximum user accessibility? Human-centred design which immerses the patient or service user in the design process to ensure design is with the whole population in mind. And systems safety assessment which proactively designs risk out of systems and avoid incidents rather than merely reactively preventing a recurrence.

An integrated approach to frame our thinking is outlined in Figure 14.1. This framework can be used as a set of activities to guide critical questions relating to people, systems, design and risk, alongside the more familiar quality improvement methodologies described in Chapter 4. In doing so, we enhance our

注重沟通、团队合作和网络社区。

展望未来，人工智能的前景是在自动化过程中嵌入持续改进，成为能够自我发展和持续改进的机器和系统。质量改进者的角色随之改变，需要与设计人工智能系统的人建立全新的关系，对其核心的决策过程和算法有深刻的理解，并有监督职能，确保所有的变革都是一种改进，无论起点如何。

系统思维

任何改进计划都需要考虑如何将我们的行动与日常临床操作和专业发展结合起来。理想情况下，目标是协调、评估、产生大的影响，以改进医疗系统实践的精确度。这涉及从系统、技术和流程的角度进行思考，其中很多都相互关联，使得任何改进工作的背景变得复杂。

使用系统方法，目的是确定最佳的服务系统设计和实施策略（英国皇家工程院，2017 年）。现有的改进方法可以通过使用系统工程中的技术来完善。其中包括包容性设计，它提出了一些重要的问题："我们服务的用户中有多大比例可以轻松访问我们提供的服务的系统？我们如何系统地设计最大的用户访问量？"以人为本进行设计，让患者或服务用户沉浸在设计过程中，以确保设计考虑到整个人群。系统安全评估，主动设计系统外的风险，避免事故发生，而不仅是被动地防止再次发生。

图 14.1 概述了构建思维框架的综合方法。这个框架可以作为一套流程来指导与人员、系统、设计和风险相关的关键问题，还包括了第 4 章中描述的更为熟悉的质量改进方法。通过这样做来提高实现有效、可持续变革的能力和效力。

capability and potency in delivering effective and sustainable change.

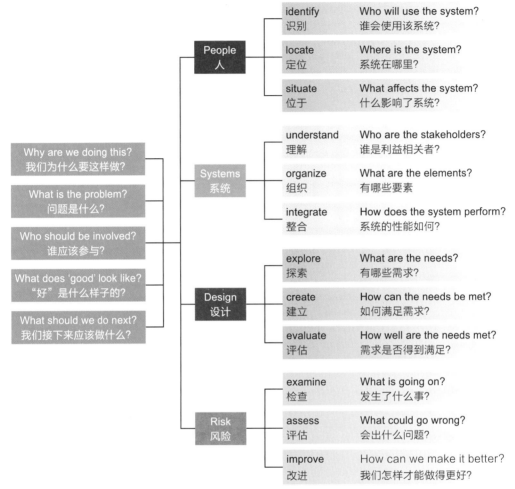

Figure 14.1 Systems thinking – key questions. Source: Royal Academy of Engineering, August 2017. Reproduced with permission

图 14.1　系统思维——关键问题。来源：英国皇家工程院，2017 年 8 月，经允许改编

Systematic learning and resilience

'A learning health care system is one in which science, informatics, incentives, and culture are aligned for continuous improvement and innovation, with best practices seamlessly embedded in the care process, patients and families active participants in all elements, and new knowledge captured as an integral by-product of the care experience.' (Institute of Medicine, 2012)

系统学习与弹性

"学习型医疗保健系统是一个将科学、信息学、激励机制和文化结合起来进行持续改进和创新的系统，将最佳实践无缝嵌入到医疗过程中，患者和家庭积极参与所有要素，并将学习新知识作为在护理过程中取得的额外收获。"（医学研究所，2012 年）

Fully embedded, integrated, systematic learning is essential as we harness technology to aid us in our improvement endeavours. Quality improvement mechanisms can play a major role in enhancing systemic learning and resilience within healthcare systems. This includes the use of clear measurement metrics and performance monitoring of service delivery across all levels of the systems, the application of proven quality improvement approaches into the processes of improving care delivery and strengthening leadership and management capacity.

Using research to study how improvement practice can get better has as an important role in developing an evidence base to our learning and how sustainable and replicable improvements to the quality of patient care can be made in healthcare more quickly. One of the live debates in improvement research is the degree to which small-scale quality improvement has value. Mary Dixon-Woods has eloquently critiqued the lack of evidence underpinning quality improvement, highlighting that 'wanting to improve is not the same as knowing how to do it'. QI is pervaded by optimism bias' (Dixon-Woods, 2019). She also describes the 'problem of many hands' with many improvement efforts being carried out in isolation, unconnected with similar initiatives elsewhere (Dixon-Woods and Pronovost, 2016). While recognising that working solely at microsystem level has its limitations, much of quality improvement work does generate significant patient and service benefits – particularly when attention is given to context. And working at small scale is a good place to start. This gives us the opportunity to learn the fundamentals of how change works, and what doesn't work. This builds our capability to scale up and spread small tests of change and align improvement efforts with wider systems of care maximising the potential for success of any improvement efforts and outputs. Systematic approaches to improvement are discussed in more detail in Chapter 4.

Leadership development

The fourth industrial revolution brings with it a need for intentional and deliberate leadership in how we manage humans (hearts and minds) and technical tools. These are not easy skills to develop, but again (and as described in Chapter 12) there is much in common with

当我们利用技术来帮助改进时，完全嵌入的、集成的、系统的学习是必不可少的。质量改进机制可以在加强医疗系统的学习和恢复能力方面发挥重要作用。这包括使用明确的测量标准和对系统各级服务提供绩效监测，将经验证的质量改进方法应用于改进护理服务的流程中，以及加强领导和管理能力。

研究改进实践如何变得更好，对于为学习建立证据基础，以及如何在医疗保健领域更快地对患者护理质量进行可持续和可复制的改进具有重要作用。小规模质量改进的价值有多大是改进研究中争论的焦点之一。玛丽·狄克森 – 伍兹雄辩地批评了缺乏支持质量改进的证据的行为，强调"想要改进并不等于知道如何去做，质量改进普遍存在乐观的偏见"（Dixon-Woods，2019 年）。她还描述了"多手问题"，许多改进工作是孤立进行的，与其他地方的类似举措没有联系（Dixon-Woods 和 Pronovost，2016 年）。虽然认识到在小型系统层面上工作有其局限性，但许多质量改进工作确实会给患者服务带来显著的好处——特别是在关注环境时。小规模改进是一个很好的起点，这让我们有机会了解变革如何起作用以及哪些不起作用，培养扩大和传播小型变革测试的能力，并使改进工作与更广泛的护理系统保持一致，从而最大限度地提高改进工作的效果的潜力。第 4 章更详细地讨论了改进的系统方法。

领导力开发

第四次工业革命的到来，使我们在管理人类（心灵和思想）和技术工具方面需要有更深远的意识。这些技能并不容易培养，但同样（如第 12 章所述）与我们如何在行动中

how we lead quality improvement in action and the skills welearn when making change happen. Encouraging alignment of purpose, methodologies and connectedness is essential. Fostering relationships and engaging others are critical. Supportive leadership focuses on valuing the viewpoint, skills and expertise of others, creating networks for connecting and collaboration, and building confidence and trust in each other. Never have these leadership skills been more needed as we navigate and strengthen the human element within physical cyber systems.

领导质量改进以及在实现变革过程中学到的技能有很多共同之处。保持目标、方法和联系的一致至关重要，培养关系和吸引他人也是至关重要的。支持型领导侧重于重视他人的观点、技能和专业知识，创建用于联系和协作的网络，以及建立彼此的信心和信任。我们在物理信息系统中漫游时，需要提高对人的关注，这些领导技能从未像现在这样迫切需要。

Sustainable health and healthcare

Beyond the impact of technology on healthcare and health-care improvement, environmental sustainability is an increasingly legitimate domain of quality improvement activity; vital, indeed, to our ability to continue to provide high - quality care into the future and to protect the health of current and future generations (Mortimer et al., 2018). A sustainable approach expands how we conceive value in healthcare to include the measurement of health outcomes against environmental and social impacts alongside financial costs (Figure 14.2).

By including these additional dimensions, there is the potential to harness our quality improvement efforts to shape a more sustainable health service, while improving patient outcomes. The 'Sustainability into Quality Improvement (SusQI)' framework shown in Box 14.1 (see also Figure 14.3) describes how a whole systems view can include scanning for environmental, social and economic resource use when mapping the current system. This allows the full range of inputs and outputs to be recognised, highlighting wastes and potential

可持续的健康和医疗保健（服务）

除了技术对医疗保健及其改进有影响之外，环境可持续性在质量改进活动中也变得越来越合理。事实上，对于我们在未来继续提供高质量护理，保证当代人及后代健康至关重要（Mortimer 等，2018 年）。可持续的方法扩展了我们对医疗保健价值的构想，包括平衡健康与环境、社会影响以及财政成本（图 14.2）。

在调理患者状况期间，这些额外的维度，以及质量改进的努力，有可能形成潜在的可持续的卫生服务。框 14.1 所示的"可持续性转化为质量改进（SusQI）"框架（另见图 14.3）描述了在映射当前系统时，整个系统如何利用环境、社会和经济资源。这样就可以确认所有的输入和输出，突出可能在改进工作的设计中被忽略的浪费和潜在收益。此外，更多地了解碳减排承诺越可能激发创造性思维，鼓励人们从根本上挑战现状。审查

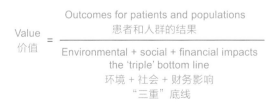

Figure 14.2 Sustainable value in healthcare. Source: Mortimer et al. (2018). Adapted with permission.

图 14.2 医疗保健的可持续价值。资料来源：莫蒂默等（2018 年），经允许改编

Box 14.1 **A framework for building sustainability into quality improvement.**
框 14.1   **将可持续性融入质量改进的框架**

QI element 质量改进要素	Sustainability content 可持续性内容	Intended benefits 预期收益
Setting goals 确定目标	Sustainability as a domain of quality; relationship to other domains 保证质量的可持续性；与其他领域的关系	New motivation to contribute to QI; energy for change 为质量改进贡献新动力；变革的能量
Studying the system 研究系统	Understanding environmental and social resource use and impacts; carbon hotspots in health services; 'seven capitals' matrix 了解环境和社会资源的使用和影响；医疗卫生服务中的碳热点；"七核心"矩阵	Highlights waste and opportunities that are often overlooked; stimulates radical thinking 强调经常被忽视的浪费和机会；激发发散思维
Designing the improvement 改进设计	Sustainable clinical practice (prevention, patient empowerment and self-care, lean systems, low carbon alternatives)[1] drivers and process changes 可持续性临床实践（预防、患者授权和自我护理、优化系统、低碳替代品）[1] 的驱动因素和流程变革	Directs towards highest value improvements, future proofing 面向具有最高价值的改进，面向未来
Measuring impact and return on investment 评估影响和投资回报	Triple bottom line/sustainable value equation; measuring carbon 三重底线 / 可持续价值方程；碳排放测量	Drives sustainable change; allows benefits to be communicated to broader audience, not exclusively regarding financial benefits 推动可持续变革；使更广泛的群众获益，而不只是考量经济效益

[1] Centre for Sustainable Healthcare (see Figure 14.3).
[1] 可持续医疗中心（图 14.3）
Source: Centre for Sustainable Healthcare (https://sustainablehealthcare.org.uk/susqi). Adapted with permission.
资料来源：可持续医疗中心 (https://sustainablehealthcare.org.uk/susqi)，经允许改编

Patient empowerment and self-care
患者自我护理

Support patients to take a biggerrole in managing their own healthand healthcare
支持患者在管理自身健康和医疗保健方面发挥更大的作用

Prevention
预防

- Promoting health
  促进健康
- Preventing disease
  预防疾病
- Reduce the need forhealthcare
  减少医疗需求

Lean service delivery
优化服务交付

- Services where people needthem
  在人们需要的地方提供服务
- Streamlining care to minimizelow value activity
  简化护理以尽量减少低价值劳动

Low carbon alternatives
采用低碳产品做替代

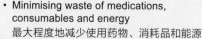

- Preferential use of effective treatment and medical technologies with lower environmental impact
  优先使用对环境影响较小的治疗方法和医疗技术
- Minimising waste of medications, consumables and energy
  最大程度地减少使用药物、消耗品和能源

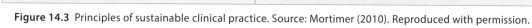

Figure 14.3 Principles of sustainable clinical practice. Source: Mortimer (2010). Reproduced with permission.
   图 14.3   可持续的临床实践原则。资料来源：莫蒂默（2010 年），经允许改编

assets that could otherwise be overlooked in the design of the improvement effort. In addition, understanding the scale of carbon reduction commitments may stimulate creative thinking and encourage people to more radically challenge the status quo. Measuring the impact of a quality improvement initiative on sustainable value is to make visible the true costs and benefits too often overlooked (such as effects on staff working conditions or patient time or carbon foot-print) at a system-wide level to inform and drive improvements in each area.

质量改进计划是否可持续，是为了在全系统范围内使人们看到经常被忽视的真实成本和收益（如对员工工作条件或患者时间或碳足迹的影响），从而获得信息，推动各个领域的改进。

Summary

Advances in digital technology, including AI, are the driving forces behind the fourth industrial revolution and how medicine is being reimagined. The pace of change is relentless and to play an effective role in this era of rapid change, skills in improvement are essential. To understand and exploit the best value from the digital world and to be able to continuously improve it are shared skills. Managing risk and uncertainty, systems thinking and systematic learning are integral competences. How we strengthen the human element is ever more important and with it the connectedness of communities and the environments which they inhabit. Equipping ourselves with these skills and behaviours in our professional development means we are better placed to play a significant and meaningful leadership role in the changing face of, and for sustainable, future health and healthcare.

总结

包括人工智能在内的数字技术的进步，是第四次工业革命以及医学如何被重新构想的驱动力。变革的步伐是无情的，要在这个快速变革的时代做出有效的贡献，提高技能必不可少。了解和利用数字世界的最大价值并能够不断改进是必备的技能，管理风险和不确定性，具备系统思维和系统学习能力不可或缺。如何突出人的因素变得越来越重要，社区居民和他们居住的环境之间的联系也随之变得更加重要。在我们的职业发展中，让自己具备这些技能和价值，意味着能够更好地在未来不断变化的健康和医疗环境中发挥重要而有意义的领导作用。

References

参考文献

Dixon-Woods M. (2019) How to improve healthcare improvement. *British Medical Journal,* 366, l5514.

Dixon-Woods M and Pronovost PJ. (2016) Patient safety and the problem of many hands. *BMJ Quality& Safety,* 25, 485-488.

Institute of Medicine (2012) *Roundtable on Value and Science-Driven Health Care,* Washington, DC, The Roundtable.

Mortimer F. (2010) The centre for sustainable healthcare principles of sustainable clinical practice. The sustainable physician. *Clinical Medicine,* 10 (2), 110-111.

Mortimer F, Isherwood J, Wilkinson A et al. (2018) Sustainability in quality improvement: redefining value. *Future Healthcare Journal,* 5, 88-93.

Royal Academy of Engineering (2017) *Engineering Better Care, A Systems Approach to Health and Care Design and Continuous Improvement.* Available at: www.raeng.org.uk/ publications/reports/engineering-better-care (accessed 7 October 2019).

World Economic Forum (2019) *Health and Healthcare in the Fourth Industrial Revolution. Insight Report.* Available at: www.weforum.org/docs/WEF_Shaping_the_Future_of_ Health_Council_Report.pdf (accessed 7 October 2019).

Further reading and resources
深度阅读与相关资源

Academy of Medical Royal Colleges (2019) Artificial Intelligence in Healthcare. Available at: www.aomrc.org.uk/reports-guidance/artificial-intelligence-in-healthcare/ (accessed 7 October 2019).

Academy of Medical Royal Colleges (2019) Training for Better Outcomes. Developing Quality Improvement into Practice. Available at: www.aomrc.org.uk/wp-content/uploads/2019/06/ Developing_QI_into_practice_0619.pdf (accessed 7 October 2019).

Castle-Clarke S. (2018) *What Will New Technology Mean for the NHS and its Patients? Four Big Technological Trends,* London, The Kings Fund.

Gray M. (2011) *How to Get Better Value Healthcare,* 2nd edn, Oxford, Offox Press.

Topol E. (2019) *Preparing the Healthcare Workforce to Deliver the Digital Future.* An independent report on behalf of the Secretary of State for Health and Social Care. Available at: https://topol.hee.nhs.uk/wp-content/uploads/HEE-Topol-Review-2019.pdf (accessed 7 October 2019).